# OSCEsmart

# 50 Medical Student OSCEs
## in Obstetrics & Gynaecology

Dr. Rochelle Brainerd

Executive Consulting Editor:
Dr. Sam Thenabadu

Ordering Information: Quantity sales. Special discounts are available on quantity purchases by corporations, associations, and others. For details, contact the publisher at the address above.

Orders by UK trade bookstores and wholesalers please visit www.scowenpublishing.com

Although every effort has been made to check this text, it is possible that errors have been made, readers are urged to check with the most up to date guidelines and safety regulations.

The authors and the publishers do not accept responsibility or legal liability for any errors in the text, or for the misuse of the material in this book.

Publisher's Cataloging-in-Publication data : OSCEsmart 50 medical student OSCEs in Obstetrics & Gynaecology

ISBN-10: 0-9985267-1-1
ISBN-13: 978-0-9985267-1-3

'For Tabitha, Bella, Ethan, Amarachi, Lily & Thea.
And Mum & Dad, always.'
**Rochelle**

'For Ammi, Molly, Reuben and Rafa - I.L.Y.T.T.M.'
**Sam**

# Contents

# Message from the authors

Doctors of all seniorities can remember the stress of the OSCE but even more so the stress of trying to study and practice for the OSCEs. A multitude of generic undergraduate and postgraduate resources can be found on line but quality, quantity, and completeness of content can vary. The aim of the OSCESmart editorial team is to bring together specialty focused books that have identified 50 core stations encompassing the essential categories of history taking, examinations, emergency moulages, clinical skills and data interpretation with a strong theme of communications running through all the stations.

The combined experience of consultants, registrars and junior doctors to write, edit and quality check these stations, promises to deliver content that is appropriate to reach a standard we would expect of new junior doctors entering their foundation internship years and into core training. It is important to know that these stations are all newly written and based at the level of clinical competencies we would expect from these grades of doctors. Learning objectives exist for undergraduate curricula and for the foundation years, and the scenarios are based and written around these. What they are not, are scenarios that have been 'borrowed' from any medical school.

Preparation is the key to success in most things, but never more so than for the OSCEs and a candidate that hasn't practised will soon be found out. These books will allow you to practice relevant scenarios with verified checklists to learn both content and the generic approach. The format will allow you to practice in groups with one person being the candidate, one the actor and one the examiner. Each scenario finishes with three learning points. Picture these as are three core learning tips that we would want you to take away if you had only a couple of days left to the exam. These OSCE scenarios promise to be a robust revision aide for the student looking to recap and consolidate for their exams, but equally importantly prepare them for life in clinical practice.

I am immensely proud of this OSCESmart series. I have had the pleasure of working with some of the brightest and most dynamic young clinicians and educators I know, and I am sure you will find this series covering the essential clinical specialties a truly robust and invaluable companion in those stressful times of revision. I must take this opportunity to thank my colleagues for all their hard work but most of all to thank my wonderful wife Molly for her unerring love and support and my sons Reuben and Rafael for all the joy they bring me.

Despite the challenging times the health service finds itself in, being a doctor remains a huge privilege. We hope that this OSCESmart series goes some way to help you achieve the excellence you and your patients deserve.

Best of luck, Dr Sam Thenabadu

# Introduction to OSCESmart in Obstetrics & Gynaecology:

Obstetrics & Gynaecology is one of few specialties that encompasses both medicine and surgery. With limited exposure at medical school, students can often find themselves merely skimming the surface of what is a complex, dynamic and critical aspect of the service provided by healthcare professionals. In a specialty rooted in asking personal questions, managing emergencies and tackling ethical dilemmas, medical students can often find themselves overwhelmed by the potential scenarios they may face in the OSCE. This book is designed to cover these topics, increasing your confidence in the period leading up to the exam.

We present a range of scenarios in Obstetrics & Gynaecology, outlining the scenarios often seen within the field. Many of the scenarios in this book have been based on real-life experiences that we have faced both as medical students and Foundation Year Doctors. This highlights the importance of achieving competence in this field, regardless of whether you intend to pursue a career in Obstetrics & Gynaecology.

The section on History Taking focuses on the specifics of discussing sensitive topics with patients, emphasising key questions that enable a clinician to differentiate between diagnoses. Whilst it is difficult to learn to perform skills from reading a book, our sections on Examinations and Explaining Skills & Procedures aim to reinforce the clinical practices that you would have developed through practical skills experience. Furthermore, it emphasises the need to explain processes and investigations without the use of medical jargon.

Clear communication and an empathetic manner are paramount for any career in medicine. Our sections on Counselling and Ethics & Law focus on the importance of effective communication, as well as the intricacies of dealing with vulnerable patients and complex situations.

This book has been created as a revision aide, enabling you to recap and revise core topics in the run-up to your examinations. The stations are designed for use in group revision sessions, with learning points highlighting the fundamental take home messages for each topic.

I sincerely hope that you find this book complements your revision in those crucial last few weeks. The best advice I can give you is to be each other's harshest critics. Some of the co-authors have been pushing me since the beginning of medical school, and others I have met along the way. I can confidently say that they have all been instrumental in getting me through both undergraduate and postgraduate exams! I am incredibly grateful for their efforts in making these scenarios as relevant and as educational as possible. Best of luck!

Rochelle Brainerd

# About the Authors

## Dr. Rochelle Brainerd
## MBBS BSc (Hons)

Dr. Rochelle Brainerd graduated from UCL Medical School in 2013 and completed her foundation training at the Royal Sussex County Hospital, Brighton and Princess Royal University Hospital, Orpington, Kent.

She has been involved in teaching throughout medical school with the UCL Target Medicine project, encouraging and supporting students from North London schools to apply to Medicine and provide equal opportunities.

During her foundation year training, she was awarded the Top Teacher Award 2014 from Brighton & Sussex Medical School and received a King's College Medical Education Award for Teaching in 2015. She has continued to develop her skills in clinical and simulation teaching and has also been an examiner for King's College London Medical School.

She is currently working as a GP trainee in North East London.

# Dr Sam Thenabadu

## MBBS MRCP DRCOG DCH MA Clin Ed FRCEM MSc (Paed) FHEA

Consultant Adult & Paediatric Emergency Medicine
Honorary Senior Lecturer & Associate Director of Medical Education

Sam Thenabadu graduated from King's College Medical School in 2001 and dual trained in Adult and Paediatric Emergency Medicine in London before being appointed a consultant in 2011 at the Princess Royal University Hospital. He has Masters degrees in Clinical Medical Education and Advanced Paediatrics.

He is undergraduate director of medical education at the King's College NHS Trust and the academic block lead for Emergency Medicine and Critical Care at King's College School of Medicine. At postgraduate level he has been the Pan London Health Education England lead for CT3 paediatric emergency medicine trainees since 2011. Academically he has previously written two textbooks and has published in peer review journals and given numerous oral and poster presentations at national conferences in emergency medicine, paediatrics, medical education and patient quality and safety.

He has an unashamed passion for medical education and strives to achieve excellence for himself, his colleagues and his patients, hoping to always deliver this through an enjoyable learning environment. Service delivery and educational need not be two separate entities, and he hopes that those who have had great teachers will take it upon themselves to do the same for others in the future.

## Co-authors

Dr. Nadir Chowdhury MBBS BSc (Hons)
ST1 Paediatrics, London
Honorary Clinical Teaching Fellow, UCL Medical School

Dr. Melania Ishak MBBS BSc (Hons)
Obstetrics & Gynaecology Trust SHO, London

Dr. Rumana Lasker MBBS BSc (Hons)
GPST1, London

Dr. Amisha Mehta MBBS BSc (Hons)
GPST2, Oxford

Dr. Shreya Morzeria MBBS BSc (Hons)
GPST1, London

Dr. Anna Rosen MBChB DRCOG
GPST1, London

Dr. Kavita Shapriya MBBS BSc (Hons) MRCP
Core Medical Trainee Year 2, London

Dr. Surenthini Suntharalingam MBBS BSc (Hons) MRCP Speciality
Registrar in Haematology, Bristol

## Abbreviations

| | |
|---|---|
| AFP | Alpha fetoprotein |
| β-hCG | human chorionic gonadotrophin beta subunit |
| BD | Twice daily |
| BMI | Body mass index |
| BNF | British National Formulary |
| BP | Blood pressure |
| CEMD | Confidential Enquiry into Maternal Deaths |
| CIN | Cervical Intraepithelial Neoplasia |
| COCP | Combined oral contraceptive pill |
| CTG | Cardiotocography |
| CVS | Chorionic venous sampling |
| DM | Diabetes mellitus |
| DVT | Deep vein thrombosis |
| ECV | External cephalic version |
| ED | Emergency Department |
| ERPC | Evacuation of retained products of conception |
| FBC | Full blood count |
| FSRH | Faculty of Sexual & Reproductive Health |
| GDM | Gestational Diabetes |
| GMC | General Medical Council |
| GP | General Practice/Practitioner |
| GUM | Genitourinary medicine |
| HELLP | Haemolysis, elevated liver enzymes and low platelets |
| HIV | Human Immunodeficiency virus |
| HPV | Human Papilloma Virus |
| HRT | Hormone replacement therapy |
| IMB | Intermenstrual bleeding |
| IUCD/IUD | Intrauterine (copper) device |
| IUGR | Intrauterine growth restriction |
| IUS | Intrauterine system |
| IV | Intravenous |
| LAM | Lactational Amenorrhoea Method |
| LARC | Long-acting reversible contraception |
| LLETZ | Large loop excision of transformation zone |

| | |
|---|---|
| LMP | Last menstrual period |
| LOA | Left occiput anterior |
| LSCS | lower segment Caesarean section |
| MSU | Mid-stream urine |
| NHS | National Health Service |
| NICE | National Institution for Clinical Excellence |
| OAB | Overactive Bladder |
| OCP | Oral contraceptive pill |
| OD | Once daily |
| OGTT | Oral glucose tolerance test |
| PCB | Post-coital bleeding |
| PCP | Pneumoncystis carinii pneumonia |
| PCOS | Polycystic ovarian syndrome |
| PEP | Post-exposure prophylaxis |
| PID | Pelvic inflammatory disease |
| PO | Per oral / orally |
| POP | Progesterone only pill |
| PPH | Postpartum haemorrhage |
| PrEP | Pre-exposure prophylaxis |
| PTSD | Post-traumatic stress disorder |
| PV | Per vaginal |
| ROA | Right occiput anterior |
| RPOC | Retained products of conception |
| SFD | Small for dates |
| STI | Sexually transmitted infection |
| TDS | Three times daily |
| TOP | Termination of pregnancy |
| USS | Ultrasound scan |
| UTI | Urinary tract infection |
| VBAC | Vaginal birth after caesarean (section) |
| WHO | World Health Organisation |

# HISTORY TAKING

## Station 1 - Dysmenorrhoea

### Candidate Instructions

You are the Foundation Year Doctor in the Gynaecology outpatient clinic. Huda is a 26-year-old woman presenting with a history of painful periods. Please take a history but you do not need to examine the patient.

After 6 minutes the examiner will stop you and ask you to summarise back your findings, suggest your management plan and answer some direct questions.

## Actor Instructions

Your name is Huda and you are a 26-year-old shop assistant. You have come to the Gynaecology outpatient clinic with a history of painful periods.

You periods started when you were 13 years old. They have always been regular – every 28 days, lasting 5-6 days with no bleeding or spotting between periods. You have not experienced any pain during sex and no bleeding after sex. You have no abnormal discharge. You have not noticed any pain when passing urine or opening your bowels. You have not experienced any rectal bleeding.

Your last period started 7 days ago. They used to be manageable, with heavy bleeding and mild cramping for the first 2 days. However, in the last 8 months, they have become very painful and have started to impact your work and social life. They are also heavier with clots and you now need to change your tampons every 3 hours on the first 2-3 days, although you have not experienced any leakage. You have been getting constant cramping lower abdominal pain radiating down your thighs, worse on days 2-3, occasionally so bad you have had to go home from work. You have tried taking Ibuprofen, which helps but wears off quickly.

You are otherwise fit and well with no other medical problems, and no recent weight loss. Your smears are up to date and have always been normal. You are in a long-term relationship and you use condoms and not tried any hormonal contraception. You have never had an STI. You have no allergies and do not take any other medication. You do not smoke and you drink 1-2 glasses of wine at weekends.

You work as a shop assistant and spend most of the day on your feet. Your boss has been understanding but struggles to find cover at short notice when you take time off. You are worried about the impact this will have on your career as you were hoping to be promoted to assistant manager this year.

You are anxious about what is causing the heavy, painful periods and you want to find a way to stop them impacting your personal and professional life.

## Examiner Instructions

The candidate is a Foundation Year Doctor in the Gynaecology outpatient clinic. They have been asked to speak to Huda, a 26-year-old woman presenting with a history of painful periods. The candidate should take a history and present their findings.

After 6 minutes, please stop the candidate and ask:

"Please summarise your findings and discuss how you would like to investigate and manage this patient."

**Mark Scheme**

| Task | Achieved | Not Achieved |
|---|---|---|
| Introduces self, washes hands | | |
| Confirms name, age & occupation of patient | | |
| Establishes reason for consultation | | |
| | | |
| Asks about menstrual history and cycle | | |
| Asks about change in periods over time | | |
| Asks about pain ("SOCRATES" approach) | | |
| Asks about associated heavy bleeding | | |
| Asks about dyspareunia, post coital bleeding, intermenstrual bleeding and vaginal discharge | | |
| Asks about non gynaecological symptoms (urinary/bowel symptoms) | | |
| Asks about weight loss or systemic features | | |
| Asks about smears, STIs and gynaecological procedures | | |
| Elicits past medical history, drug and allergy history | | |
| Elicits social and family history | | |
| Asks about treatment offered so far and impact on symptoms | | |
| Identifies patient's ideas, concerns and expectations in an empathetic manner | | |
| | | |
| Summarises history in clear and concise manner | | |
| Suggests appropriate differentials (e.g. fibroids, adenomyosis, endometriosis) | | |
| Suggests appropriate examination and investigation (FBC, USS) | | |
| Suggests appropriate management options | | |
| Completes station in a confident and professional manner | | |
| | | |
| Examiners Global Mark | /5 | |
| Actors Global Mark | /5 | |
| Total Station Mark | /30 | |

4

## Learning points

- Do not forget to ask about the impact on the patient's social and professional life. This will often guide patient's expectations of your management plan.

- Primary dysmenorrhea is diagnosed *after* excluding any organic cause, and is most common at menarche

- It is important to ask about the *progression* of symptoms, as your likely differentials would change depending on how the patient's symptoms have evolved over time.

# Station 2 - Menorrhagia

## Candidate Instructions

You are the Foundation Year Doctor in the Gynaecology outpatient clinic. Celeste is a 34-year-old woman presenting with a history of heavy menstrual bleeding. Please take a history but you do not need to examine the patient.

After 6 minutes the examiner will stop you and ask you to summarise back your findings, suggest your management plan and answer some direct questions.

# Actor Instructions

Your name is Celeste and you are a 34-year-old social worker. You have come to the Gynaecology outpatient clinic today with heavy periods.

For the last 10 months, you have noticed you periods are much heavier and more uncomfortable - still every 30 days, but now lasting 7-8 days instead of 4 days previously. You regularly pass clots, and have had some embarrassing experiences when you have leaked onto the bedding and through your clothes. You change your pads every 1-2 hours at times.

Your periods started when you were 12 years old. You have not experienced any bleeding between periods or after sex, and no pain during sex. You have no abnormal discharge. You have not experienced any excessive bruising, prolonged bleeding or nosebleeds. Your smears are up to date and have always been normal. You have never had as STI. You are married and use condoms with your husband. You had a miscarriage at seven weeks in 2013 and had 1 other pregnancy with a 5-year-old daughter but would like to have more.

You have no medical problems and no allergies. You have been feeling increasingly tired, especially around your periods. Your GP started you on Tranexamic Acid 2 months ago to which has been helpful but you are still having leaks. He also found you are anaemic and started you on iron supplements. You were not keen to start hormonal treatment as you were worried about how it would affect your body in the long run.

You do not smoke or drink alcohol. You moved to the UK from Ghana 15 years ago and you live with your husband and daughter and work as a social worker. Your mother also suffered with heavy periods but you are not sure why.

You are anxious to find out why you are bleeding so much and how to stop this, as you no longer socialise during your periods because you are scared of flooding. It is also causing problems with your husband as you are now having sex less often as your periods are longer.

## Examiner Instructions

The candidate is a Foundation Year Doctor in the Gynaecology outpatient clinic. They have been asked to speak to Celeste, a 34-year-old woman presenting with a history of heavy periods. The candidate should take a history and present their findings.

After 6 minutes, please stop the candidate and ask:

"Please summarise your findings and discuss how you would like to investigate and manage this patient."

**Mark Scheme**

| Task | Achieved | Not Achieved |
|---|---|---|
| Introduces self, washes hands | | |
| Confirms name, age & occupation of patient | | |
| Establishes reason for consultation | | |
| | | |
| Asks about menstrual history and cycle | | |
| Asks about change in periods over time | | |
| Asks about symptoms of anaemia | | |
| Asks about symptoms/signs of clotting abnormalities | | |
| Asks about dyspareunia, post coital bleeding and intermenstrual bleeding | | |
| Asks obstetric history | | |
| Asks about contraception, smears, STIs and gynaecological procedures | | |
| Asks about weight loss or systemic features | | |
| Elicits past medical history, drug and allergy history | | |
| Elicits social and family history – asks about impact on social life | | |
| Asks about treatment offered so far and impact on symptoms | | |
| Identifies patient's ideas, concerns and expectations in an empathetic manner | | |
| | | |
| Summarises history in clear and concise manner | | |
| Suggests appropriate differentials (e.g. fibroids) | | |
| Suggests appropriate examination and investigation (Bloods, USS) | | |
| Suggests appropriate management options – medical and surgical according to history | | |
| Completes station in a confident and professional manner | | |
| | | |
| Examiners Global Mark | /5 | |
| Actors Global Mark | /5 | |
| Total Station Mark | /30 | |

## Learning points

- It is important to identify the impact that symptoms have on the patient's day-to-day life, as this is key to managing their expectation of your treatment plan.

- Note that in the history, the patient was unsure of the long-term effects of hormone therapy. Giving the patient information and picking up on their concerns could make them more willing to accept hormonal treatment options, which can be very effective in the management of menorrhagia.

- Establish whether the patient is trying to conceive or not or if they would like to in the future, as this would impact the appropriate management options. Many of the surgical treatment options can impact on fertility so careful counseling is important.

# Station 3 - Oligomenorrhoea

## Candidate Instructions

You are the Foundation Year Doctor in the Gynaecology outpatient clinic. Anisa is a 19-year-old woman who has presented with irregular periods. Please take a history but you do not need to examine the patient.

After 6 minutes the examiner will stop you and ask you to summarise back your findings, suggest your management plan and answer some direct questions.

## Actor Instructions

Your name is Anisa, and you are a 19-year-old student. You have presented to the Gynaecology clinic with a long history of irregular periods.

You started having periods when you were 14 years old and they have always been irregular. You frequently miss periods and have had a total of 7 periods in the last 12 months. They last for 4-5 days with mild cramps and are not particularly heavy, and you do not get any bleeding between periods. Your last period was 19 days ago. You are not sexually active and state that you never have been.

You are otherwise fit and well apart from suffering with acne for which you use benzoyl peroxide gel, although this has not helped after 4 months. You are also generally quite hairy but you put this down to your ethnicity as it also affects your family. You also tend to get stubborn chin hairs and dark underarms. You are on no other medication and have no allergies.

You also struggle with your weight but are trying to eat more healthy food now that you are living in student halls and cooking for yourself. Your BMI is 26 (overweight). You drink alcohol socially and have never smoked. Your mum also had irregular periods and your younger sister, Hanna, is due to have an ultrasound scan as she is yet to start her period. She recently turned 17 years old.

Your GP suggested starting tablets but you declined, as you wanted more investigations to find out what is wrong. You are concerned about your symptoms after finding out your sister is being investigated and are worried that you may need a scan as well.

## Examiner Instructions

The candidate is a Foundation Year Doctor in the Gynaecology clinic. They have been asked to speak to Anisa, a 19-year-old woman who has presented with irregular periods. The candidate should take a history and present their findings.

After 6 minutes, please stop the candidate and ask:

"Please summarise your findings and discuss how you would like to investigate and manage this patient."

## Mark Scheme

| Task | Achieved | Not Achieved |
|---|---|---|
| Introduces self, washes hands | | |
| Confirms name, age & occupation of patient | | |
| Establishes reason for consultation | | |
| | | |
| Asks about duration of symptoms | | |
| Specifically identifies if symptoms have been present since menarche or developed later on | | |
| Asks about menstrual history and cycle | | |
| Asks about signs or symptoms of hyperandrogenism (hirsutism, acne, hair loss) | | |
| Asks about signs or symptoms of insulin resistance (acanthosis nigricans, obesity) | | |
| Elicits full gynaecological history (IMB, PCB, dyspareunia) | | |
| Establishes risk of pregnancy or STI with sexual history if relevant | | |
| Elicits past medical history, drug & allergy history | | |
| Elicits social history and family history | | |
| Asks about emotional or physical stress | | |
| Identifies patient's ideas, concerns and expectations in an empathetic manner | | |
| Enquires about treatment offered so far | | |
| | | |
| Summarises history in clear and concise manner | | |
| Suggests likely diagnosis of PCOS | | |
| Suggests appropriate examination & investigations (bloods, USS) | | |
| Suggests management options | | |
| Completes station in a confident and professional manner | | |
| | | |
| Examiners Global Mark | /5 | |
| Actors Global Mark | /5 | |
| Total Station Mark | /30 | |

## Learning points

- Think about polycystic ovary syndrome (PCOS) with irregular, infrequent periods or infertility. However, do not forget to exclude pregnancy or STIs.

  Polycystic ovaries are very common on ultrasound and up to 33% of reproductive age woman may have them. A small proportion of this group actually has PCOS. Insulin resistance e.g. central obesity or acanthosis nigricans, is not part of the diagnostic criteria but can be an indirect sign of PCOS. The Rotterdam diagnostic criteria *(Rotterdam ESHRE/ASRM-Sponsored PCOS Consensus Workshop Group, 2003)* requires 2 of the following 3:

    - Polycystic ovaries (either 12 or more peripheral follicles or increased ovarian volume (greater than 10 cm$^3$).
    - Oligo-ovulation or anovulation.
    - Clinical and/or biochemical signs of hyper-androgenism.

- Do not forget to ask about smears if the patient is over 25 years of age. In the UK women are invited for cervical screening between the ages of 25 and 64 (*Public Health England, 2015*). Women aged 25–49 are invited every three years and women aged 50–64 are invited every five years.

## Station 4 - Amenorrhoea

## Candidate Instructions

You are the Foundation Year Doctor at a GP practice. Elena is a 21-year-old woman who has presented with problems with her periods. Please take a history but you do not need to examine the patient.

After 6 minutes the examiner will stop you and ask you to summarise back your findings, suggest your management plan and answer some direct questions.

# Actor Instructions

Your name is Elena, and you are a 21-year-old university student reading graphic design. You have presented to your GP with concerns about your periods.

You have not had a period for the last 4 months. Your periods used to be regular and never caused you any problems before. If specifically asked, you had your first period at the age of 14. You had a regular 28-day cycle, and the bleeding would typically last 3-4 days. You were worried you may be pregnant so took a pregnancy test about 3 months ago. This was negative and you have not been sexually active since. If asked, your last sexual encounter was 3.5 months ago with your ex-partner, and you used condoms.

You have found that you are more stressed lately about a number of things. Firstly, as this is the final year of your degree, you have a big design project due in 6 months. You also split up with your partner recently, whom you had been with since the start of university. In order to deal with the stress, you have been going to the gym more, and typically work out 7 days a week from 5-6am, as well as having dance rehearsals 4 times a week. You have noticed have lost approximately 3kg. You had a progress check at the gym last week and they calculated your BMI from your height and weight as being 18 and noted this was 'underweight'.

You have not noticed any change to your hair growth, and no other systemic symptoms such as headaches, upon questioning.

You have no other medical history, and are not on any medications. You do not smoke or drink alcohol. You have been pregnant once 2 years ago and had a medical termination at 6 weeks. You had chlamydia, which was treated 3 years ago and have had a clear STI screen 2 months ago.

You are extremely anxious to find out why your periods have suddenly stopped as you feel this is only adding to your stresses – please press the candidate to offer suggestions for causes of this. You are worried this is because you had a termination and now you will never have kids. You are hoping that your GP could suggest why you may be having this problem and send you for some tests.

## Examiner Instructions

The candidate is a Foundation Year Doctor in a GP surgery. They have been asked to speak to Elena, a 21-year-old woman who has presented with problems with her periods. The candidate should take a history and present their findings.

After 6 minutes, please stop the candidate and ask:

"Please summarise your findings and discuss how you would like to investigate and manage this patient."

**Mark Scheme**

| Task | Achieved | Not Achieved |
|---|---|---|
| Introduces self, washes hands | | |
| Confirms name, age & occupation of patient | | |
| Establishes reason for consultation | | |
| | | |
| Asks about duration of symptoms | | |
| Asks about menstrual history and cycle prior to onset of amenorrhoea | | |
| Asks about presence of associated symptoms of menstrual cycle e.g. pelvic pain | | |
| Asks about current emotional or physical stress | | |
| Asks specifically about exercise pattern | | |
| Elicits obstetric history/prior pregnancies | | |
| Elicits gynaecological and brief sexual history – establishes risk of STIs | | |
| Establishes risk of current pregnancy | | |
| Elicits past medical history, drug & allergy history | | |
| Elicits social history and family history | | |
| Identifies patient's ideas, concerns and expectations in an empathetic manner | | |
| Can suggest possible causes and reassures patient that it is likely due to reversible causes | | |
| | | |
| Summarises history in clear and concise manner | | |
| Suggests likely diagnosis of secondary amenorrhoea due to stress and exercise | | |
| Suggests appropriate examination & investigations (bloods, USS) | | |
| Suggests management options | | |
| Completes station in a confident and professional manner | | |
| | | |
| Examiners Global Mark | /5 | |
| Actors Global Mark | /5 | |
| Total Station Mark | /30 | |

## Learning points

- It is important to establish early on if this is primary or secondary amenorrhoea in order to tailor your questions to identify the likely cause. *Primary* amenorrhoea is the failure to reach menarche by 16 years of age. *Secondary* amenorrhoea describes the cessation of periods for 6 months or more in a woman who has previously had normal menstrual cycles.

- Remember the old proverb that will always save your neck: any woman of childbearing age is pregnant until proven otherwise!

- Consider endocrine causes of amenorrhoea and the associated symptoms to consider in your history taking if appropriate.

# Station 5 - Taking a Sexual History

## Candidate Instructions

You are the Foundation Year Doctor in the Emergency Department. Martha is a 24-year-old woman who has presented with lower abdominal pain and discharge. Please take a focused gynaecological and sexual history. You do not need to examine the patient.

After 6 minutes the examiner will stop you and ask you to summarise back your findings, suggest your management plan and answer some direct questions.

# Actor Instructions

Your name is Martha, and you are a 24-year-old student doing your Masters in Journalism. You have presented to the Emergency Department with lower abdominal pain that started 4 days ago, and is now 6-7/10 in severity if asked. It is a constant dull ache and does not move anywhere, does not get better/worse throughout the day or with any positions although Ibuprofen has helped a little. You feel nauseous and sweaty, and you have no urinary or bowel symptoms.

You have not noticed any abnormal vaginal bleeding but have seen some yellowish/green frothy discharge. You have taken the COCP for contraception for the last 3 years, and have light, relatively painless bleeds for 5 days during the break. You have not noticed any bleeding after sex but occasionally do notice that it can be painful during penetration, which has been intermittent for the past 2-3 months, but you have not mentioned this to your GP.

Three months ago, you changed sexual partners and had an STI check where you were found to have chlamydia. The nurse practitioner at the clinic gave you given a week-long course of treatment, however you did not complete this as you were concerned it would interfere with the pill and you are worried about getting pregnant. You have not had any other sexual partners since then. If asked, you have had 3 male sexual partners in the last 6 months, and had a combination of oral, anal and vaginal sex, occasionally unprotected with all three. You have had 1 previous episode of chlamydia treated 2 years ago. You are not aware of any partners having HIV or Hepatitis or being IV drug users, and you have never used drugs. You had a negative HIV test at the clinic 3 months ago.

You have not been offered a smear test yet. You got pregnant once last year, which ended in a medical termination at 7 weeks, but you would like to have children in the future.

You are otherwise well with mild asthma managed with a salbutamol inhaler when required. You have no allergies. You live in a flat share while doing your Masters. You have no other relevant family history.

You are concerned this could all be because you did not complete the treatment from the STI clinic, and if the possibility of pelvic inflammatory disease is explained, you are very concerned that this may mean you will not be able to have children in the future.

## Examiner Instructions

The candidate is a Foundation Year Doctor in the Emergency Department. They have been asked to speak to Martha, a 24-year-old woman who has presented with lower abdominal pain and discharge. The candidate should take a focused gynaecological and sexual history and present their findings.

After 6 minutes, please stop the candidate and ask:

"Please summarise your findings and discuss how you would like to investigate and manage this patient."

**Mark Scheme**

| Task | Achieved | Not Achieved |
|---|---|---|
| Introduces self, washes hands | | |
| Confirms name, age & occupation of patient | | |
| Establishes reason for consultation | | |
| | | |
| Asks thorough history of pain ("SOCRATES" approach) and associated symptoms | | |
| Asks about vaginal discharge | | |
| Asks about urinary or bowel symptoms | | |
| Asks about other systemic symptoms | | |
| Takes full gynae history (IMB, PCB, dyspareunia) | | |
| Elicits obstetric history/prior pregnancies/TOPs | | |
| Gives warning shot re. sensitive questions and reiterates confidentiality | | |
| Asks about sexual partners in last 6 months: gender, type of sex and contraceptive use | | |
| Asks about high risk behaviour for HIV/Hepatitis | | |
| Asks about previous and current STIs and completion of treatment | | |
| Elicits past medical history, drug & allergy history | | |
| Identifies patient's ideas, concerns and expectations in an empathetic manner | | |
| | | |
| Summarises history in clear and concise manner | | |
| Suggests likely diagnosis of PID but *highlights* ectopic pregnancy to be excluded | | |
| Suggests examination & investigations – *highlights* ectopic must be excluded first | | |
| Suggests management options & appropriate antibiotics | | |
| Completes station in a confident and professional manner | | |
| | | |
| Examiners Global Mark | /5 | |
| Actors Global Mark | /5 | |
| Total Station Mark | /30 | |

# Learning points

- Pelvic inflammatory disease (PID) is a general term for infection of the upper female genital tract, including the uterus, fallopian tubes, and ovaries. Risk factors for PID include multiple previous sexual partners, young age (<30), lack of barrier contraception, termination of pregnancy or miscarriage, and an IUCD inserted within the last 20 days.

- Look over current guidelines for appropriate treatment of common STIs, as well as PID. This can occasionally be managed in the community but if severe, the patient should be admitted.

- It is important to be sensitive and non-judgemental when discussing sexual history. Patients can often feel embarrassed and stigmatised as a result of this diagnosis. As their doctor, it is important to make them feel comfortable to open up so you can treat them quickly and appropriately.

# Station 6 - Vaginal discharge

## Candidate Instructions

You are the Foundation Year Doctor in a GP surgery. Fiona is a 23-year-old woman presenting with vaginal discharge. Please take a focused history from her but you do not need to examine the patient.

After 6 minutes the examiner will stop you and ask you to summarise back your findings, suggest your management plan and answer some direct questions.

## Actor Instructions

Your name is Fiona, and you are a 23-year-old actress. You have come to see your GP today as you noticed a whitish discharge in your underwear for the past week. When asked, describe the discharge as thick and lumpy, which is odourless. You first thought it was normal vaginal discharge but became concerned when it got heavier. The discharge is associated with itchiness and redness around the vulva. You have also noticed some discomfort passing urine, but no change in the colour or smell.

The candidate should ask you about your sexual history, and if they do not give a warning shot, act surprised and embarrassed. You are heterosexual and are currently sexually active. You are currently in a relationship and have been with your partner for 3 months. You have had a total of 2 sexual partners in the last 6 months. You have only had intercourse with your current partner in the last 3 months.

You had an STI check at the start of this relationship, which was negative, and you have never had an STI before. You have no other symptoms. You are currently on the combined oral contraceptive pill. You do not use condoms with your partner, and if comfortable, you confide that you are worried that you might have a sexually transmitted infection as you have had concerns that your partner has been unfaithful.

You have never been pregnant. You have regular 'normal' periods, with no intermenstrual bleeding or pain or bleeding during or after sex. If asked, you have no relevant past medical history, and you have no allergies. There is no relevant family history. You do not smoke and do not drink alcohol.

Please press the candidate for what they think is the most likely diagnosis, citing that you are concerned that your partner has been sleeping around.

## Examiner Instructions

The candidate is a Foundation Year Doctor in a GP surgery. They have been asked to speak to Fiona, a 23-year-old woman presenting with a history of vaginal discharge. The candidate should take a focused history and present their findings.

After 6 minutes, please stop the candidate and ask:

"Please summarise your findings and discuss how you would like to investigate and manage this patient."

**Mark Scheme**

| Task | Achieved | Not Achieved |
|---|---|---|
| Introduces self, washes hands | | |
| Confirms name, age & occupation of patient | | |
| Establishes reason for consultation | | |
| | | |
| Asks about colour and consistency of discharge | | |
| Asks about odour of discharge | | |
| Asks about local skin changes or pruritus | | |
| Asks about urinary symptoms | | |
| Asks about dyspareunia, post coital bleeding, intermenstrual bleeding and vaginal discharge | | |
| Gives warning shot re. sensitive questions and reiterates confidentiality | | |
| Elicits full sexual history | | |
| Asks about contraceptive use | | |
| Asks about last STI check and smear test | | |
| Elicits obstetric and gynaecological history | | |
| Elicits past medical history, drug & allergy history | | |
| Identifies patient's ideas, concerns and expectations in an empathetic manner | | |
| Reassures patient that this is unlikely to be an STI | | |
| Suggests appropriate diagnosis (candidiasis) | | |
| Suggests appropriate examination and investigation | | |
| Suggests appropriate management plan (i.e. topical Clotrimazole, PO Fluconazole) | | |
| Completes station in a confident and professional manner | | |
| | | |
| Examiners Global Mark | /5 | |
| Actors Global Mark | /5 | |
| Total Station Mark | /30 | |

## Learning points

- Sexual history still remains a difficult topic for many patients to discuss. They are often embarrassed or scared, and therefore a sensitive and empathetic approach is essential. Always start with a warning shot and reiterate confidentiality. It is important though not to let your own embarrassment make you cut corners. These lines of questioning should be conducted in as thorough a manner as you would for any medical history taking.

- It is worth looking over the differences in vaginal discharge in terms of colour, odour and associated symptoms as different presentations may indicate different aetiologies and thus are managed differently.

- Remember to think about the patient's concerns. The history points towards thrush, a very treatable condition that is not sexually transmitted. Addressing these concerns could potentially realign her thought process and take away unnecessary stress on her relationship.

# Station 7 - Urinary Incontinence

## Candidate Instructions

You are the Foundation Year Doctor in the Urogynaecology outpatient clinic. Audrey is a 57-year-old woman presenting with a history of urinary incontinence. Please take a history but you do not need to examine the patient.

After 6 minutes the examiner will stop you and ask you to summarise back your findings, suggest your management plan and answer some direct questions.

## Actor Instructions

Your name is Audrey, a 57-year-old supermarket worker. You have come to the Urogynaecology clinic with a 1-year history of intermittent urinary incontinence which has progressively worsened.

You tend to leak small amounts of urine when coughing, sneezing and laughing. On a few occasions, you have not been able to hold your bladder and wet yourself, which was incredibly upsetting. This can occur at any time of the day and with no warning, meaning you now tend to wear bulky sanitary pads every time you go out to avoid another embarrassing incident.

You have not experienced urinary frequency, bloody urine, pain or waking through the night to urinate. You tend to run to the toilet as soon as you get to the front door but have occasionally had some accidents. You have a good stream when you do pass urine. You have not had a heavy sensation in your vagina or noticed any lumps externally. Your bowels are normal and are not hard to pass, and you have not been incontinent of stools. You have not had pelvic pain or bloating and you have had no vaginal bleeding or discharge.

You have 3 children. The first delivery was quite traumatic with forceps, and the other 2 were normal vaginal deliveries with no complications. You reached the menopause 5 years ago. You have Type 2 Diabetes and Hypertension and you have struggled with your weight all your life – you currently weigh 85kg and have gained about 8kg this year. Your BMI is currently 34. You currently take Metformin 500mg TDS and Amlodipine 5mg OD. You have no allergies.

You are married and live with your husband, and you are infrequently sexually active. You work at the till and rarely exercise. You have smoked 10 cigarettes/day since you were 18. You do not drink alcohol but currently have 6-7 cups of tea a day.

So far, you have tried pelvic floor exercises advised by your GP, but often forget to do these and you are wondering if there is some kind of pill that can make things better, fast.

You are concerned as your symptoms are getting worse and affecting your work. You have started to avoid social engagements and visiting unfamiliar places, as you are worried about having an accident.

## Examiner Instructions

The candidate is a Foundation Year Doctor in the Urogynaecology clinic. They have been asked to speak to Audrey, a 57-year-old woman presenting with a history of urinary incontinence. The candidate should take a history and present their findings.

After 6 minutes, please stop the candidate and ask:

"Please summarise your findings and discuss how you would like to investigate and manage this patient."

**Mark Scheme**

| Task | Achieved | Not Achieved |
|---|---|---|
| Introduces self, washes hands | | |
| Confirms name, age & occupation of patient | | |
| Establishes reason for consultation | | |
| | | |
| Asks about duration & progression of symptoms | | |
| Differentiates between symptoms of stress or urge incontinence | | |
| Asks about activities precipitating incontinence (e.g. lifting, straining, coughing) | | |
| Asks about urinary symptoms to exclude UTI | | |
| Asks about nocturia and stream of urine | | |
| Asks about symptoms of prolapse/fistula | | |
| Specifically asks about sensation (or lack of) when passing urine | | |
| Asks about bowel symptoms/incontinence | | |
| Elicits obstetric and gynaecological history | | |
| Elicits past medical history, drug & allergy history | | |
| Elicits social history and family history | | |
| Identifies patient's ideas, concerns and expectations in an empathetic manner | | |
| | | |
| Summarises history in clear and concise manner | | |
| Identifies type of urinary incontinence | | |
| Suggests appropriate examination and investigation (Bloods, USS) | | |
| Suggests appropriate management options – conservative, medical and surgical | | |
| Completes station in a confident and professional manner | | |
| | | |
| Examiners Global Mark | /5 | |
| Actors Global Mark | /5 | |
| Total Station Mark | /30 | |

## Learning points

- Stress incontinence is due to sphincter incompetence and leads to release of small amounts of urine when intra-abdominal pressure is increased. It may also be associated with genitourinary prolapse. The management of this is different to urge incontinence, where there is detrusor instability or hyperreflexia leading to an involuntary detrusor contraction. These phenomena may be idiopathic or secondary to neurological problems. Inevitably it is important to identify which is the key issue affecting the patient in order to manage appropriately.

- Do not forget to ask about the impact of symptoms on the patient's day-to-day life. The severity of symptoms can also determine the most suitable management options for the patient.

- Cystoscopy is not recommended in the investigation of women where incontinence is the only presenting complaint. A range of urodynamic studies exist to provide objective information regarding the normal and abnormal function of the urinary tract and pelvic floor and, therefore, a better understanding of the cause of symptoms.

# Station 8 - Subfertility

## Candidate Instructions

You are the Foundation Year Doctor in the Gynaecology outpatient clinic. Ellie is a 34-year-old woman who has been referred by her GP for difficulty conceiving. Please take a history but you do not need to examine the patient.

After 6 minutes the examiner will stop you and ask you to summarise back your findings, suggest your management plan and answer some direct questions.

## Actor Instructions

Your name is Ellie, and you are a 34-year-old teacher. You and your partner of 5 years, James, have been trying to conceive for the past 1 year. You try to have unprotected sex 3-4 times a week but you are both becoming quite stressed with work and with the lack of success in getting pregnant and so it is not always possible.

You have never been pregnant although James has 2 young children from a previous relationship. (Try to steer the candidate away from questions about your partner.)

You started having periods at age 13, and they were initially irregular but you now have a 30-day cycle and bleed for 5 days. This is always very heavy and very painful and has actually been getting worse. The pain can often start 1-2 days before your period actually starts. You have no pain during sex, after sex or between periods. Your smears are up to date and always normal and you have never had an STI.

You have no issues with your weight, and you do not have problems with excess hair growth, acne or nipple discharge.

You previously used the depot injection but stopped 2 years ago. You have no other medical issues aside from an appendectomy when you were 14 years old. You currently take folic acid in preparation for pregnancy. You have no other allergies. If asked about family history, you recall that your mother may have also had heavy, painful periods but she is now well into the menopause.

You are concerned that you will never be able to have children. James tries to reassure you but you are worried he will leave you and you keep pushing him away, which is causing friction in your relationship. You work as a teacher, which is also very stressful. Home and work has been so difficult that you reluctantly admit you have started smoking 5 cigarettes a day again after stopping 2 years ago.

## Examiner Instructions

The candidate is a Foundation Year Doctor in the Gynaecology clinic. They have been asked to speak to Ellie, a 34-year-old woman who has been referred by her GP for difficulty conceiving. The candidate should take a history and present their findings.

After 6 minutes, please stop the candidate and ask:

"Please summarise your findings and discuss how you would like to investigate and manage this patient."

**Mark Scheme**

| Task | Achieved | Not Achieved |
|---|---|---|
| Introduces self, washes hands | | |
| Confirms name, age & occupation of patient | | |
| Establishes reason for consultation | | |
| | | |
| Asks about duration of difficulty conceiving | | |
| Asks about previous conception or pregnancies | | |
| Asks if male partner has been able to conceive with other women | | |
| Asks about frequency of intercourse | | |
| Asks about systemic symptoms and signs (galactorrhoea, hair growth, weight) | | |
| Asks about smears and STIs | | |
| Asks about stress and effect on relationship | | |
| Asks specifically about menstrual cycle | | |
| Elicits full gynaecological history | | |
| Elicits past medical history, drug & allergy history | | |
| Elicits social history and family history | | |
| Identifies patient's ideas, concerns and expectations in an empathetic manner | | |
| Summarises history in clear and concise manner | | |
| Suggests differentials (endometriosis, fibroids, idiopathic subfertiliy) | | |
| Suggests appropriate examination & investigations of both partners | | |
| Suggests management options or follow up | | |
| Completes station in a confident and professional manner | | |
| | | |
| Examiners Global Mark | /5 | |
| Actors Global Mark | /5 | |
| Total Station Mark | /30 | |

## Learning points

- History is pertinent here especially with respect to factors that directly impact fertility and those which do so indirectly, such as previous contraceptive choice, previous abdominal surgery and stress.

- Always consider male subfertility. In this scenario, the partner has been able to successfully conceive twice. Despite this, it is still important to take a full history from the male partner to identify areas of concern. Drugs and alcohol can reduce male fertility, as well as infections, anatomical abnormalities and antisperm antibodies.

- Positive evidence-based information can encourage an anxious couple. For example, 80% of couples will conceive within a year and 90% within two years, providing the woman is under 40 years old and they are having regular intercourse (*NICE, Aug 2016*). Fertility issues can be difficult to discuss and can often impact on a patient's self esteem and relationship. It is important to deal with this sensitively and explore the effects it is having on her personal life.

# Station 9 - Vaginal Bleeding in Early Pregnancy

## Candidate Instructions

You are the Foundation Year Doctor in the Early Pregnancy Assessment Unit. Louise is a 25-year-old woman who is 7 weeks pregnant. She has attended today with a history of vaginal bleeding. Please take a focused history but you do not need to examine the patient.

After 6 minutes the examiner will stop you and ask you to summarise back your findings, suggest your management plan and answer some direct questions.

## Actor Instructions

Your name is Louise, and you are a 25-year-old receptionist. You have presented to the Early Pregnancy Assessment Unit with spotting in the past few days. You are currently 7 weeks pregnant with your first pregnancy and you and your partner Tom are overjoyed.

Two days ago you noticed some blood on wiping, but you have noticed that it has since been more noticeable with a 50p size amount of fresh red blood present on your knickers. You have not noticed any clots. You have also had some mild crampy central abdominal pain today radiating down and is currently 4/10 severity if asked. You have not noticed any shoulder tip pain. You have been feeling nauseous today and vomited after a light breakfast but thought it could just be morning sickness. You have felt sweaty today, but not felt dizzy or light headed.

You found out you were pregnant 2 weeks ago and your last period was 7 weeks ago. You have been trying to get pregnant for 18 months and finally managed to get pregnant naturally. You had chlamydia when you were 19 but this was treated at the time. You have had no abnormal discharge, and you were previously on the COCP but stopped 18 months ago. You have never has a smear.

You are otherwise well and not on any medication aside from folic acid. You have no known allergies. You live with your partner and work as a receptionist. You do not smoke or drink. You have no relevant family history.

You are very concerned that you are having a miscarriage as you have been trying for such a long time – please press the candidate for an explanation or confirmation of this. You really want an urgent scan so you can reassure yourself that the baby is ok.

# Examiner Instructions

The candidate is a Foundation Year Doctor in the Early Pregnancy Assessment Unit. They have been asked to speak to Louise, a 25-year-old woman who has presented with lower abdominal pain and discharge. The candidate should take a focused history and present their findings.

After 6 minutes, please stop the candidate and ask:

"Please summarise your findings and discuss how you would like to investigate and manage this patient."

**Mark Scheme**

| Task | Achieved | Not Achieved |
|---|---|---|
| Introduces self, washes hands | | |
| Confirms name, age & occupation of patient | | |
| Establishes reason for consultation | | |
| | | |
| Asks about history of bleeding including quantity, appearance and duration | | |
| Asks about abdominal pain ("SOCRATES") | | |
| Asks about shoulder tip pain | | |
| Asks about nausea | | |
| Asks about other systemic symptoms | | |
| Takes full gynae history (IMB, PCB, dyspareunia) | | |
| Elicits obstetric history/prior pregnancies/TOPs | | |
| Establishes dates of current pregnancy & LMP | | |
| Asks about history of STIs | | |
| Asks about smear tests | | |
| Elicits past medical history, drug & allergy history | | |
| Elicits brief social and family history | | |
| Identifies patient's ideas, concerns and expectations in an empathetic manner | | |
| | | |
| Summarises history in clear and concise manner | | |
| Suggests suitable differentials including ectopic, miscarriage or appendicitis | | |
| Suggests examination & investigations – *highlights* that ectopic must be excluded | | |
| Suggests management options | | |
| Completes station in a confident and professional manner | | |
| | | |
| Examiners Global Mark | /5 | |
| Actors Global Mark | /5 | |
| Total Station Mark | /30 | |

# Learning points

- Always exclude an ectopic pregnancy before anything else. Missing this can be devastating for the pregnant woman's health and fertility. All symptomatic pregnancies should be considered as possible ectopics until a scan has confirmed an inter-uterine pregnancy, as the management of these patients will be far more aggressive, mostly with inpatient scanning. Young women with ectopics can appear very well right up to the point of rupturing.

- It is important to manage this woman's concerns and expectations appropriately. She is clearly most concerned about the possibility of miscarrying, with the significant majority of miscarriages occurring in the first trimester. The medical term for 'miscarriage' is 'spontaneous abortion' (if <24 weeks gestation) however in lay terms, this often implies a conscious termination of the pregnancy so language should be used diplomatically.

- Consider non-gynaecological causes as well – a urinary tract infection or even appendicitis are very realistic differentials in this scenario.

# Station 10 - Abdominal Pain in Early Pregnancy

## Candidate Instructions

You are the Foundation Year Doctor in the Emergency Department. Harriet is an 18-year-old woman who is 11 weeks pregnant and has presented with abdominal pain. Please take a history but you do not need to examine the patient.

After 6 minutes the examiner will stop you and ask you to summarise back your findings, suggest your management plan and answer some direct questions.

## Actor Instructions

Your name is Harriet, and you are an 18-year-old sales assistant. You have presented to the Emergency Department complaining of lower abdominal pain for the past 3 days. You are currently 11 weeks pregnant with your first baby.

If asked specifically, the pain started as a dull 'tummy ache' and was constant in the middle of your tummy, but now is more noticeable on the right side and is currently 7/10 severity and sharp. It is worse when getting up or if you touch it. You have been feeling generally unwell, lost your appetite and have felt hot. You have not opened your bowels in 2 days, but not had any diarrhoea. You have no urinary symptoms. You have been getting morning sickness, which usually settles by midday but you have noticed it has lasted all day since the pain has come on. You have had no bleeding or spotting and not noticed any vaginal discharge or itching.

This is your first and only pregnancy and has so far been unremarkable – although you had a scare at 7 weeks with spotting and had an ultrasound that confirmed a viable uterine pregnancy. You have no other medical problems aside from Polycystic Ovarian Syndrome. You are only taking folic acid and have no other allergies. You have been with your boyfriend for 1 year and are living with him and your mum, and he has been supportive despite this being an unplanned pregnancy. You have not had any other sexual partners in the past 6 months, your last STI check was clear. You are a non-smoker and do not drink.

You are worried that you could be having a miscarriage.

## Examiner Instructions

The candidate is a Foundation Year Doctor in Emergency Department. They have been asked to speak to Harriet, an 18-year-old woman who has presented with abdominal pain and is 11 weeks pregnant. The candidate should take a history and present their findings.

After 6 minutes, please stop the candidate and ask:

"Please summarise your findings and discuss how you would like to investigate and manage this patient."

**Mark Scheme**

| Task | Achieved | Not Achieved |
|---|---|---|
| Introduces self, washes hands | | |
| Confirms name, age & occupation of patient | | |
| Establishes reason for consultation | | |
| | | |
| Asks about pain symptoms ("SOCRATES" approach) | | |
| Asks about gynae symptoms - bleeding, discharge, post coital bleeding, dyspareunia | | |
| Asks about urinary symptoms | | |
| Asks about bowel symptoms | | |
| Asks about nausea, vomiting and appetite | | |
| Asks about other systemic symptoms | | |
| Elicits obstetric history/prior pregnancies/TOPs | | |
| Asks brief sexual history and risk of STIs | | |
| Elicits past medical history, drug & allergy history | | |
| Elicits brief social history | | |
| Identifies patient's ideas, concerns and expectations in an empathetic manner | | |
| Summarises history in clear and concise manner | | |
| Suggests suitable differentials including miscarriage, ovarian pathology or appendicitis | | |
| Suggests examination & investigations | | |
| Recognises urgency of excluding serious differentials e.g. torsion, appendicitis | | |
| Suggests management options | | |
| Completes station in a confident and professional manner | | |
| | | |
| Examiners Global Mark | /5 | |
| Actors Global Mark | /5 | |
| Total Station Mark | /30 | |

## Learning points

- Keep PID in mind – this is a young female who has had an unplanned pregnancy eluding to likely unprotected sexual intercourse with infective symptoms – make sure you consider this when thinking of how to investigate.

- Abdominal pain in pregnancy must always make you consider ectopic pregnancies. Fortunately this lady has had a scan confirming an intra-uterine pregnancy. It is not impossible to have both an intra and extra uterine (heterotropic) pregnancy with rates of approximately 1:30 000 for natural conceptions and significantly higher of 1-3:100 for assisted conceptions (*Kirk E., Bottomley C., Bourne T., 2013*), however the scan should identify both.

- Do not forget non O&G causes! The gynaecological symptoms are a red herring in this case. Keep an open mind when thinking of differentials for common problems – pregnant women are more prone to having a range of conditions including appendicitis, pancreatitis, cholecystitis, pyelonephritis to name but a few. A collaborative approach with the emergency physician, gynaecologist and surgeon may be required in the first instance.

# Station 11 - Pruritus in Pregnancy

## Candidate Instructions

You are the Foundation Year Doctor in the General Obstetrics Clinic. Natalie is a 27-year-old woman who is 30 weeks pregnant and has been referred by her GP due to ongoing pruritus. Please take a history but you do not need to examine the patient.

After 6 minutes the examiner will stop you and ask you to summarise back your findings, suggest your management plan and answer some direct questions.

## Actor Instructions

Your name is Natalie, and you are a 27-year-old lawyer. You have been referred by your GP to the General Obstetrics Clinic with uncontrollable itching. You are currently 30 weeks pregnant with your second baby.

You have experienced itching over the past two weeks and it is gradually getting worse. If asked specifically, it is affecting the palms and soles more than anywhere else, but is also noticeable on your tummy and legs. At first, you thought it would get better on its own and so you left it for a week and moisturised daily. However, as it became more intense, you went to your GP and he referred you here.

You have not noticed any yellowing of your skin or eyes. You have had no abdominal pain or change to your urine or stools. You feel well in yourself with no fevers, sweats or headaches and do not feel confused. You have not had a rash per se, but have redness from intense itching.

There has been no change in washing powder, soaps or creams. You have not started any new medications or taken anything over the counter. Nobody else you have been in contact with has experienced similar symptoms.

You have no significant past medical history. You take no regular medications and have no known allergies. You have no relevant family history. You live with your husband and two daughters aged 6 & 8 who are all fit and well. Both girls were normal vaginal deliveries at full term without complications. You have had no other pregnancies or gynaecological symptoms.

You are a non-smoker and used to drink 2-3 glasses of wine a week prior to getting pregnant.

Your main concern is finding out what is causing this intense itching as it is really impacting on your quality of life and you are worried it could be something serious. You are constantly thinking about it and your skin is starting to become sore from all the scratching. You would like to know if there are any medications that may help with the symptoms.

## Examiner Instructions

The candidate is a Foundation Year Doctor in the General Obstetrics Clinic. They have been asked to speak to Natalie, a 27-year-old woman who has been referred by her GP due to ongoing pruritus. The candidate should take a history and present their findings.

After 6 minutes, please stop the candidate and ask:

"Please summarise your findings and discuss how you would like to investigate and manage this patient."

**Mark Scheme**

| Task | Achieved | Not Achieved |
|---|---|---|
| Introduces self, washes hands | | |
| Confirms name, age & occupation of patient | | |
| Establishes reason for consultation | | |
| | | |
| Asks about duration of symptoms | | |
| Asks about specific locations of itching | | |
| Asks about presence of rash with itching | | |
| Asks about jaundice or change in colour of urine or stools | | |
| Asks about other systemic symptoms | | |
| Asks about environmental changes (e.g. detergent, clothing, dust) | | |
| Asks about changes to medication including over the counter remedies | | |
| Asks about effect on daily life | | |
| Elicits current and previous obstetric history | | |
| Elicits past medical history, drug & allergy history | | |
| Elicits social history & family history | | |
| Identifies patient's ideas, concerns and expectations in an empathetic manner | | |
| Summarises history in clear and concise manner | | |
| Suggests suitable differentials | | |
| Suggests examination & investigations (bloods, USS abdomen) | | |
| Suggests management options according to differentials e.g. ursodeoxycholic acid | | |
| Completes station in a confident and professional manner | | |
| | | |
| Examiners Global Mark | /5 | |
| Actors Global Mark | /5 | |
| Total Station Mark | /30 | |

## Learning points

- Do not forget to ask about sites of pruritus – this is often a key indicator to the diagnosis. Obstetric cholestasis often affects the palms and soles, whereas Polymorphic Eruption of Pregnancy and Prurigo of Pregnancy often affect the abdomen and limbs.

- Always consider pemphigoid gestationis, which is rare but can have serious complications such as IUGR and prematurity. It is characterised by a blistering vesicular rash and should be managed as a high risk pregnancy

- Do not forget to consider other non-pregnancy related causes, including liver, renal or haematological disease.

# Station 12 - Antepartum Haemorrhage

## Candidate Instructions

You are the Foundation Year Doctor in the Maternity Triage Unit. Kiran is a 27-year-old woman who is 32 weeks pregnant and has presented with vaginal bleeding. Please take a history but you do not need to examine the patient.

After 6 minutes the examiner will stop you and ask you to summarise back your findings, suggest your management plan and answer some direct questions.

## Actor Instructions

Your name is Kiran, and you are a 27-year-old bank manager. You have presented to the Maternity Triage Unit with vaginal bleeding since yesterday. You are currently 32 weeks pregnant with your first baby.

Yesterday, you noticed some light spotting with fresh red blood. You tried not to panic as you had sexual intercourse the night before and thought it may be due to this. Today, the bleeding has been heavier and you noticed your pad was quite significantly stained today so decided to come to the hospital. You also noted a sharp 'twinge' in your lower belly this afternoon when you had heavier bleeding, although this has now settled. You have not noticed any vaginal discharge and have not had a rush or trickle of fluid. You felt the baby moving lots mainly in the morning but it has been quieter this afternoon, which you put down to the baby being asleep.

You have not had any episodes of bleeding in this pregnancy until now and it has otherwise been uneventful. If directly asked, your 20-week scan showed a 'low-lying placenta' but the sonographer advised you this was quite common.

Your first and only other pregnancy was 5yrs ago and you gave birth to a healthy girl. The pregnancy was normal but you had an emergency caesarean for failure to progress and fetal distress. You intend on having a vaginal birth (VBAC), which the midwives have been happy with.

You last had a smear 2 years ago and it was normal. You have never had an STI, and your husband is your only sexual partner. You are otherwise fit and well. You have no regular medications and no allergies.

You do not smoke or drink alcohol. You work in a bank, which can be quite stressful. You live with your husband and daughter. You are all very excited to have a new addition to the family and you feel well supported by your partner and family.

You are very concerned about the bleeding and worried that the baby is in danger or might be premature. You are very anxious that having sex may have harmed the baby and you blame yourself.

## Examiner Instructions

The candidate is a Foundation Year Doctor in the Maternity Triage Unit. They have been asked to speak to Kiran, a 27-year-old woman who has presented with vaginal bleeding and is 32 weeks pregnant. The candidate should take a history and present their findings.

After 6 minutes, please stop the candidate and ask:

"Please summarise your findings and discuss how you would like to investigate and manage this patient."

# Mark Scheme

| Task | Achieved | Not Achieved |
|---|---|---|
| Introduces self, washes hands | | |
| Confirms name, age & occupation of patient | | |
| Establishes reason for consultation | | |
| | | |
| Asks about bleeding: quantity, colour, duration of symptoms | | |
| Asks about associated pain | | |
| Asks about other associated PV discharge/fluid | | |
| Asks about fetal movements | | |
| Asks about precipitating abdominal or vaginal trauma, including sexual intercourse | | |
| Asks about other systemic symptoms | | |
| Asks about current pregnancy including complications and scans | | |
| Elicits obstetric history and brief sexual history, including risk of STIs | | |
| Elicits past medical history, drug & allergy history | | |
| Elicits brief social history and enquires about home situation (e.g. domestic violence) | | |
| Identifies patient's ideas, concerns and expectations in an empathetic manner | | |
| | | |
| Summarises history in clear and concise manner | | |
| Suggests suitable differentials including placenta praevia or placental abruption | | |
| Suggests abdominal and PV examination | | |
| Suggests appropriate investigations to determine maternal and fetal wellbeing | | |
| Suggests management plan – admit & observe, CTG, consider steroids, anti-D if Rhesus negative | | |
| Completes station in a confident and professional manner | | |
| | | |
| Examiners Global Mark | /5 | |
| Actors Global Mark | /5 | |
| Total Station Mark | /30 | |

## Learning points

- Read the vignette carefully. This asks you to 'take a history' so do not forget to cover all aspects including past medical, drug and social history and not get carried away with just the antenatal history. As pregnancies progress, pre-existing medical issues can come to the forefront so it is important to be thorough in your history taking.

- The main causes of antepartum haemorrhage should be revised. Placenta praevia is more common in this case because of the previous Caesarean section. This defines the insertion of the placenta, partially or fully, in the lower segment of the uterus but may remain asymptomatic during the pregnancy. Placental abruption, on the other hand, is premature separation of a normally placed placenta.

- Make note of the risk of vaginal or abdominal trauma, which may not always be accidental. Domestic violence commonly presents for the first time in pregnancy, so do give the patient an opportunity to discuss this.

# Station 13 - Postpartum Haemorrhage

## Candidate Instructions

You are the Foundation Year Doctor in a GP practice. Layla is a 34-year-old woman who has presented with vaginal bleeding 10 days after giving birth. Please take a focused history but you do not need to examine the patient.

After 6 minutes the examiner will stop you and ask you to summarise back your findings, suggest your management plan and answer some direct questions.

## Actor Instructions

Your name is Layla, and you are a 34-year-old make up artist. You have presented to your GP with ongoing vaginal bleeding 10 days after giving birth.

You had quite a stressful delivery of your first baby, as it ended in an emergency caesarean for fetal distress. You had a temperature a few hours before your caesarean, and so you were given 24 hours of antibiotics. The caesarean was otherwise straightforward with no complications and you had a healthy baby girl. You were discharged 7 days ago.

You are now 10 days post delivery, and whilst you have been struggling with post-operative pain, you are mostly concerned about the continued heavy bleeding. Whilst you understand it is normal to bleed for 4-7 days post delivery, you were told it should be getting lighter and yet it is consistently heavy. You are currently changing your pad every 2-3 hours and passing clots and what appears to be dark blood. You have no offensive discharge. You have generalised lower abdominal pain and the scar site hurts every time you move.

You have a supportive partner and your mother has been at home with you. You feel generally nauseated and have had a reduced appetite since the birth. You have not had any fevers but have been having cold sweats. There are no urinary symptoms. Your bowels have been sluggish throughout the pregnancy and have not yet improved.

You have had no other pregnancies and no significant gynaecological history, and have never previously had significantly heavy periods.

You wish to know whether this bleeding is normal or if there is anything you need to be concerned about.

## Examiner Instructions

The candidate is a Foundation Year Doctor in a GP practice. They have been asked to speak to Layla, a 34-year-old woman who has presented with vaginal bleeding 10 days after giving birth. The candidate should take a focused history and present their findings.

After 6 minutes, please stop the candidate and ask:

"Please summarise your findings and discuss how you would like to investigate and manage this patient."

**Mark Scheme**

| Task | Achieved | Not Achieved |
|---|---|---|
| Introduces self, washes hands | | |
| Confirms name, age & occupation of patient | | |
| Establishes reason for consultation | | |
| | | |
| Asks about bleeding: quantity, colour, duration of symptoms | | |
| Asks about associated pain | | |
| Asks about other associated PV discharge/fluid | | |
| Asks about urinary or bowel symptoms | | |
| Asks about other systemic symptoms inc. fever | | |
| Asks about scar – e.g. discharge, oozing, open | | |
| Asks about delivery and perioperative complications | | |
| Elicits obstetric history | | |
| Elicits past medical history, drug & allergy history | | |
| Elicits brief social history | | |
| Identifies patient's ideas, concerns and expectations in an empathetic manner | | |
| | | |
| Summarises history in clear and concise manner | | |
| Recognises this as secondary PPH | | |
| Suggests suitable differentials e.g. endometritis, retained products | | |
| Suggests appropriate examination and investigations | | |
| Suggests management plan – refer, antibiotics | | |
| Completes station in a confident and professional manner | | |
| | | |
| Examiners Global Mark | /5 | |
| Actors Global Mark | /5 | |
| Total Station Mark | /30 | |

# Learning points

- Primary postpartum haemorrhage (PPH) is loss of blood estimated to be >500ml from the genital tract, within 24 hours of delivery. A minor PPH is blood loss up to 1000mls and a major PPH is >1000mls. The causes are remembered by the 4 T's – **T**one (uterine atony), **T**rauma (laceration of the uterus, cervix or vagina), **T**issue (retained placenta) and **T**hrombin (pre existing clotting issues)

- Secondary PPH occurs between 24hrs and 6 weeks post partum, and can occur in approximately 2% of spontaneous vaginal deliveries (*RCOG, 2013*). It remains the most common cause of postnatal morbidity between days 2-10. The two main causes are endometritis and retained products of conception (RPOC) (either a blood clot or retained placenta).

- The vast majority of patients with endometritis resolve within 72 hours. If the patient does not improve after a course of antibiotics, an USS +/- evacuation of retained products of conception (ERPC) is required.

# Station 14 - Puerperal Pyrexia

## Candidate Instructions

You are the Foundation Year Doctor in a GP practice. Winona is a 32-year-old woman who has presented feeling generally unwell 5 days after giving birth. Please take a history but you do not need to examine the patient.

After 6 minutes the examiner will stop you and ask you to summarise back your findings, suggest your management plan and answer some direct questions.

## Actor Instructions

Your name is Winona, and you are a 32-year-old optician, currently on maternity leave. You have presented to your GP feeling unwell for the past 24 hours with a fever.

You noted your temperature was 38.3 at home this morning but did not want to take Paracetamol as you are breastfeeding.

You gave birth 5 days ago and you were discharged home after 1 day. You gave birth to a healthy baby girl called Sammie, who is your first child. You have had no other pregnancies. The pregnancy was uncomplicated with normal antenatal scans. You went into labour at $39^{+2}$ weeks when your waters spontaneously broke at home. You came into hospital and delivered normally on the midwife led unit after 16 hours of labour. You had a small tear during the labour that did not require stitching but has been a little sore. You are passing a small amount of fresh blood vaginally but this is now much less. You have not noticed any discharge or smell.

You have been breastfeeding Sammie. At first it was going well but the last 2 days your right breast in particular has become very tender and the nipple is cracked. The breast is redder and hotter than the left. You have not noticed any rashes elsewhere.

You have been eating and drinking well until yesterday when you started to feel unwell. You have no nausea or vomiting. You have had no pain when urinating, frequency or change in colour/smell. Your bowels are opening daily with no diarrhoea. You have no cough or coryzal symptoms.

You have no past medical history and no regular medications or allergies. You have never smoked and only drink alcohol occasionally, but that was before you were pregnant. You live with your husband and new baby and are currently enjoying your maternity leave.

You should specifically ask if taking medications such as Paracetamol and antibiotics will harm Sammie and if you can continue breastfeeding.

## Examiner Instructions

The candidate is a Foundation Year Doctor in a GP practice. They have been asked to speak to Winona, a 32-year-old woman who has presented feeling generally unwell 5 days after giving birth. The candidate should take a focused history and present their findings.

After 6 minutes, please stop the candidate and ask:

"Please summarise your findings and discuss how you would like to investigate and manage this patient."

**Mark Scheme**

| Task | Achieved | Not Achieved |
|---|---|---|
| Introduces self, washes hands | | |
| Confirms name, age & occupation of patient | | |
| Establishes reason for consultation | | |
| | | |
| Asks about fever – duration, if measured, response to antipyretics | | |
| Asks about associated PV discharge/lochia | | |
| Asks about urinary or bowel symptoms | | |
| Asks about other systemic symptoms & pain | | |
| Asks about breastfeeding or breast symptoms | | |
| Asks about pregnancy, delivery and obstetric history | | |
| Elicits past medical history, drug & allergy history | | |
| Elicits brief social history | | |
| Identifies patient's ideas, concerns and expectations in an empathetic manner | | |
| Picks up on patient concerns regarding Paracetamol while breastfeeding | | |
| Reassures patient it is safe to continue breastfeeding while being treated for mastitis | | |
| | | |
| Summarises history in clear and concise manner | | |
| Recognises likely diagnosis of mastitis | | |
| Suggests suitable differentials e.g. vaginal wound infection, endometritis | | |
| Suggests appropriate examination (check uterus, IV sites, breast, legs) and investigations | | |
| Suggests suitable management plan – *highlights* need to exclude sepsis | | |
| Completes station in a confident and professional manner | | |
| | | |
| Examiners Global Mark | /5 | |
| Actors Global Mark | /5 | |
| Total Station Mark | /30 | |

## Learning points

- Pick up on cues given by the actor. The patient mentions that she is concerned about taking Paracetamol while breastfeeding – which is known to be safe in pregnancy. Use this as an opportunity to educate the patient. Additionally there are many antibiotics that are deemed safe whilst breastfeeding. A simple way to remember is that if you would give the antibiotic to the child directly it is safe to be exposed to via breastfeeding.

- Consider all causes of surgical or hospital acquired infections – check IV sites, legs for a possible DVT, chest as well as breast, uterine and PV infections.

- Maternal sepsis (in particular genital tract sepsis) remains one of the top five causes of maternal mortality in the last UK Confidential Enquiry into Maternal Deaths (CEMD) (*Nair & Knight, 2015*). Examine the patient thoroughly in order to exclude sepsis, but do not forget to 'safety net' appropriately.

# Station 15 - Postnatal Check

## Candidate Instructions

You are the Foundation Year Doctor in a GP practice. Yee is a 29-year-old woman who has come in for her 6 weeks after giving birth. Please complete her 6-week postnatal check.

You do not need to examine the patient, although please describe to the examiner what you wish to assess. You do not need to assess the baby.

After 6 minutes the examiner will stop you and ask you to summarise back your findings, suggest your management plan and answer some direct questions.

## Actor Instructions

Your name is Yee, and you are a 29-year-old pharmacist, currently on maternity leave. You have presented to your GP for your 6-week postnatal check. Your baby, Ella, has already had her 6-week check, which was normal.

You delivered 6 weeks ago at 37 weeks. You used gas and air during a normal vaginal delivery. It was quite traumatic for you as you had an episiotomy and had stitches; so sitting has been painful but has improved in the last few weeks. The health visitor reassured you it is healing well but you still have some discomfort when sitting for a long time. You are no longer experiencing any bleeding or discharge and have not noticed an offensive smell. You have not started your periods yet.

You are opening your bowels normally and passing urine but noticed you have small accidents when you laugh or cough. This is a concern as you do not want to continue wearing pads all the time, especially since the post-delivery discharge has now stopped.

You are currently fully breastfeeding and have no pain or problems with milk production. Ella has been gaining weight as expected and you are bonding well. You intend to fully breastfeed until at least 6 months. Your mood is generally quite good, apart from being very tired as you try to sleep train your baby (unsuccessfully). Your husband is very supportive but is about to start back at work full time so you will be on your own. You are anxious about this but have a good support network of friends and family nearby.

You plan to use condoms for contraception but have not had sex yet as you still feel a bit sore down below.

You have no other medical problems and are not on any medications and do not have any allergies. You do not smoke or drink alcohol. You currently live with your husband Simon and Ella.

Your main concern is the urinary incontinence when you are out and about, especially as you will be left on your own with the baby. As a result you have not made many trips out of the house, which is making you feel a bit isolated.

## Examiner Instructions

The candidate is a Foundation Year Doctor in a GP practice. They have been asked to speak to Yee, a 29-year-old woman who has attended the practice for her 6-week postnatal check. The candidate should complete the postnatal check and report to the examiner what they would like to examine and assess. They do not need to assess the baby.

After 6 minutes, please stop the candidate and ask them to present their findings and detail what they would like to assess to complete the postnatal check if they have not covered this already.

**Mark Scheme**

| Task | Achieved | Not Achieved |
|------|----------|--------------|
| Introduces self, washes hands | | |
| Confirms name, age & occupation of patient | | |
| Establishes reason for consultation | | |
| | | |
| Asks about delivery and any complications | | |
| Asks about post delivery – wound healing/pain | | |
| Asks about PV discharge, bleeding (including if menstrual cycle has resumed) or lochia | | |
| Asks about urinary and bowel symptoms, including incontinence | | |
| Asks about type of feeding and any issues | | |
| Asks about breast soreness/infective symptoms | | |
| Asks about sleeping pattern | | |
| Asks about mood and emotional issues | | |
| Asks about social support available to patient | | |
| Asks about sexual activity and contraception | | |
| Discusses contraceptive options if breastfeeding | | |
| Takes brief medical, drug, allergy and social history | | |
| Identifies patient's ideas, concerns and expectations in an empathetic manner | | |
| | | |
| Summarises history in clear and concise manner | | |
| Suggests appropriate examination of abdomen and vaginal stitches | | |
| Suggests suitable management or follow up | | |
| Completes station in a confident and professional manner | | |
| | | |
| Examiners Global Mark | /5 | |
| Actors Global Mark | /5 | |
| Total Station Mark | /30 | |

## Learning points

- The 6-week postnatal check should cover physical, psychological and social health. It is an important time to screen for any signs of mental illness, which is relatively common in the postnatal period. It is also not restricted to depression, so consider other possibilities such as anxiety and PTSD.

- Ask about bowel or urinary incontinence as a third of women experience urinary incontinence after childbirth[7] but many feel too embarrassed to bring it up themselves. Regular pelvic floor exercises are a good way for patients to manage the symptoms as first-line option.

- Always enquire about contraception and intercourse. The Lactational Amenorrhoea Method (LAM) can be effective, but only in the first 6 months, if totally amenorrhoeic, and if *fully* breastfeeding at least 4 hourly during the day and 6 hourly at night. If these three criteria are not met, additional contraception is required. After 6 weeks postpartum, fertility may return if breastfeeding reduces or stops.

# Station 16 - Postmenopausal Bleeding

## Candidate Instructions

You are the Foundation Year Doctor in the Gynaecology Clinic. Christine is a 72-year-old woman who has presented with a 2-month history of intermittent vaginal bleeding. Please take a history but you do not need to examine the patient.

After 6 minutes the examiner will stop you and ask you to summarise back your findings, suggest your management plan and answer some direct questions.

## Actor Instructions

Your name is Christine, and you are a 72-year-old retired bookkeeper. You have presented to the Gynaecology Clinic with a 2-month history of intermittent vaginal bleeding.

This is not normal for you and you have not had any bleeding of this kind since you went through menopause at 54. The bleeding is not profuse - if asked to describe the amount it is roughly the size of a 50p maybe 2-3 times a week. You have taken to wearing sanitary pads again as it is so unpredictable. The amount is increasing slightly. The blood is not fresh red but rather dark. There is no other vaginal discharge and no unusual smell. There is no pain. You are not sexually active and have not noticed any particular vaginal dryness. There is no blood in the stool or in the urine. Your bowel and urinary habits are normal. You have not had any recent weight loss.

You went through the menopause at the age of 54, having started periods at 12 years old. You were never able to have children – the cause of this was never discovered and you had not used contraception. You had regular periods throughout these years – a 28-day cycle and then bleeding for 5 days. You started going through the change in your early 50s and had significant trouble with night sweats and hot flushes. You were on a HRT tablet for 5 years. You always went for your smears and these were always normal.

Your past medical history includes a gall bladder removal when you were 35, as well as high blood pressure but this has been well controlled. Your only medication is Amlodipine 5mg. You have no allergies. You are a smoker – 15 a day for about 50 years. You do not drink alcohol. You are not aware of any relevant family history.

You are concerned because the symptoms are persisting and getting worse – you had hoped it would resolve by itself. Your friend said you might be at risk of cancer.

## Examiner Instructions

The candidate is a Foundation Year Doctor in the Gynaecology clinic. They have been asked to speak to Christine, a 72-year-old woman who has presented with a history of 2 months of PV bleeding. The candidate should take a focused history and present their findings.

After 6 minutes, please stop the candidate and ask:

"Please summarise your findings and discuss how you would like to investigate and manage this patient."

# Mark Scheme

| Task | Achieved | Not Achieved |
|---|---|---|
| Introduces self, washes hands | | |
| Confirms name, age & occupation of patient | | |
| Establishes reason for consultation | | |
| | | |
| Asks about bleeding: onset, timing, amount | | |
| Asks about associated pain | | |
| Asks about associated PV discharge or dryness | | |
| Asks about urinary or bowel symptoms | | |
| Asks about other systemic symptoms | | |
| Asks about onset of menopause | | |
| Asks about previous hormone therapy (contraception or HRT) | | |
| Elicits obstetric and gynaecological history including smears | | |
| Elicits past medical history, drug & allergy history | | |
| Elicits social and family history | | |
| Identifies patient's ideas, concerns and expectations in an empathetic manner | | |
| | | |
| Summarises history in clear and concise manner | | |
| Suggests appropriate differentials *including* endometrial cancer | | |
| Suggests examination and investigations including ultrasound | | |
| Suggests need for pipelle biopsy or hysteroscopy if abnormal or further concerns | | |
| Suggests suitable management or follow up | | |
| Completes station in a confident and professional manner | | |
| | | |
| Examiners Global Mark | /5 | |
| Actors Global Mark | /5 | |
| Total Station Mark | /30 | |

## Learning points

- Postmenopausal bleeding is endometrial cancer until proven otherwise. Differentials include atrophic vaginitis and other cancers of the female reproductive tract.

- Risk factors for endometrial cancer mainly revolve around exposure to oestrogen. The OCP and pregnancy are protective while early menarche, late menopause, nulliparity and unopposed HRT are risk factors.

- It is always important to address the patients concerns and ideas but more so in this case, as you are considering a diagnosis of cancer. It would be wrong to ignore the concerns regarding cancer, especially if they bring it up. However, discussing it as a differential diagnosis does not mean you committing to this as the final diagnosis. This takes time and practice to undertake but is an important skill to consider from an early stage.

# Explaining Skills & Procedures

## Station 17: Consenting for Cervical Smear

### Candidate Instructions

You are the Foundation Year Doctor in a GP practice. Kyra is a 25-year-old woman who is due to have her first cervical smear and has booked a double appointment. Please explain the procedure in order to take verbal consent and discuss any concerns she may have.

You do not need to examine the patient or demonstrate the procedure.

You have eight minutes.

## Actor Instructions

Your name is Kyra, and you are 25-year-old postal worker. You have presented to the GP surgery after receiving a letter to attend for your smear test. You are quite nervous and so have booked a double appointment with the doctor. You would like to know what the procedure involves and why it is important. If it is described as a 'screening' programme, ask more about what this is.

You are currently not sexually active but have been in the past. Explain this to the candidate and ask if it is still necessary to have the examination.

Your last period was 14 days ago and you have not had any bleeding, discharge or pain. You have no known medical problems, you are not on any regular medications and you have no known allergies. You smoke 5 cigarettes a day.

You are quite nervous about the procedure as you have heard some horror stories from your friends. The doctor should be sensitive to these concerns and reassuring.

If asked for questions:
- What if there are abnormalities? Will that mean I have cancer?

## Examiner Instructions

The candidate is a Foundation Year Doctor in a GP surgery. They have been asked to speak to Kyra, a 25-year-old woman who is due to have her first cervical smear and has booked a double appointment. The candidate should explain the procedure in order to take verbal consent and discuss any concerns she may have.

The candidate has been informed they do not need to examine the patient or demonstrate the procedure.

**Mark Scheme**

| Task | Achieved | Not Achieved |
|---|---|---|
| Introduces self, washes hands | | |
| Confirms name, age & occupation of patient | | |
| Establishes reason for consultation | | |
| | | |
| Establishes prior knowledge of cervical smear – why it is done and what it involves | | |
| Explains that it is a screening test for cervical cancer and explains what 'screening' is | | |
| Identifies who falls under the screening criteria | | |
| Explains what the results of the test can be | | |
| Explains what will need to be done if the tests are abnormal | | |
| Explains what treatment can be done if there are abnormal cells | | |
| Checks understanding of information given | | |
| | | |
| Offers/informs of presence of chaperone | | |
| Explain what a speculum is and insertion | | |
| Explain that a brush will be used inserted and turned three times | | |
| Explains that sample will be sent to the lab and results directly by post | | |
| Explain risks of procedure | | |
| Explain benefits of procedure | | |
| Identifies patients ideas, concerns & expectations in an empathetic manner | | |
| | | |
| Reassures patient that they will stop if in too much discomfort or changes her mind | | |
| Checks understanding (asks patient to summarise) and obtains verbal consent | | |
| Completes station in a confident and professional manner | | |
| | | |
| Examiners Global Mark | /5 | |
| Actors Global Mark | /5 | |
| Total Station Mark | /30 | |

# Learning points

- Understand how to clearly explaining what a screening programme is without the use of jargon. Patient information websites offer simple explanations that are worth reading over.

- Cervical smears are offered to women aged 25-64 at 3 yearly intervals until age 49 and then 5 yearly intervals till age 64. Certain patient groups require more frequent smears or colposcopy — i.e. HIV patients and renal transplant patients.

- It is now well known that human papillomavirus (HPV) causes the vast majority of cases of cervical cancer. In the UK and many developed countries, the HPV vaccine has been introduced for girls aged 12-13 but it will be many years before an impact on incidence of cervical cancer may be truly seen.

# Station 18: How to put on a Condom

## Candidate Instructions

You are the Foundation Year Doctor in the sexual health clinic. Adam is an 18-year-old man who has presented for the fifth time in 2 months after unprotected sex and concerns about STIs. Please explain how to put on a condom and discuss his concerns.

You do not need to take a full sexual history from this patient.

You have eight minutes.

## Actor Instructions

You are Adam, an 18-year-old computer science student in your 1st year at university. You have attended the sexual health clinic five times over the past two months after having unprotected sex.

You admit you have only had sex once before university and are not very confident putting on a condom. You also had a reaction to the condom on that occasion but you thought this was because it was free at a student party – the shop bought ones are so expensive.

You are worried about the risk of STIs and pregnancy. You attended sexual health lessons at school but do not remember the details and just want a refresher.

You are currently not in a formal relationship and are heterosexual. You are otherwise fit and well with no drug allergies. You had a rash when you used latex gloves during an experiment at school.

If the candidate does not answer the following, please ask these questions at 6 minutes.

- "How does a condom work? Do I still need to wear one if my partner is on the pill?"
- "Do I need to wear a new condom each time we have sex?"
- "What should I do if I think the condom split?"

## Examiner Instructions

The candidate is a Foundation Year Doctor at a sexual health clinic. They have been asked to speak to Adam, an 18-year-old man who has presented for the 5th time in 2 months after unprotected sex and concerns about STIs. They have been asked to explain how to put on a condom and discuss his concerns or questions.

They are not required to take a full sexual history.

## Mark Scheme

| Task | Achieved | Not Achieved |
|---|---|---|
| Introduces self, washes hands | | |
| Confirms name, age & occupation of patient | | |
| Establishes reason for consultation | | |
| | | |
| Establishes prior knowledge/use of condoms and reasons behind lack of use | | |
| Explains condoms are 'barrier' contraception – the pill does not protect against STIs | | |
| Explains efficacy – 98% (2 women pregnant per year with perfect use) | | |
| Explains can protect against *most* STIs | | |
| Establishes if patient has a latex allergy and advises regarding using latex-free condoms | | |
| | | |
| Explains how to check condom packet – kite sign, expiry date, check for tears | | |
| Explains/shows how to open and position the condom - teat facing up | | |
| Explains how to squeeze air from 'teat' area before rolling down an erect penis. | | |
| Explains must be used during all penetration | | |
| Advises to use a new condom if applied inside out as pre-seminal fluid may be on the tip. | | |
| Explains that a new condom needs to be used for each time the patient has sex | | |
| Explains what to do if there are any concerns regarding efficacy: (e.g. split, expired) | | |
| Explains can get condoms for free from clinic | | |
| Identifies patients ideas, concerns & expectations in an empathetic manner | | |
| | | |
| Summarises key points, checks understanding, offers leaflet | | |
| Maintains non judgemental approach | | |
| Completes station in a confident and professional manner | | |
| Examiners Global Mark | /5 | |
| Actors Global Mark | /5 | |
| Total Station Mark | /30 | |

# Learning points

- This station may seem simple but make note of the distribution of marks. It is important to consider all information that needs to be given and use the allocated time wisely. A non-judgemental and professional approach is key as conveying the key messages and directions will be far easier if you have the trust and confidence of the patient.

- Some universities will often have models to demonstrate with – practice this beforehand on clinical skills models.

- With explaining stations, take care to break information down into small chunks and check understanding before you move along. Large volumes of information can be difficult to digest so take care not to overwhelm patients.

# Station 19: Obtaining a Mid-stream Urine Sample

## Candidate Instructions

You are the Foundation Year Doctor at a GP practice. Tamara is a 47-year-old woman who has been experiencing dysuria, frequency and abdominal pain. She has already completed a course of antibiotics for a urinary tract infection (UTI) with little improvement. Please take a brief, focused history and explain how to obtain a midstream urine sample. Please answer any questions she may have. You do not need to examine the patient.

You have eight minutes.

## Actor Instructions

You are Tamara, a 47-year-old paramedic. You have been experiencing ongoing dysuria, frequency and lower abdominal pain for the past week. You had a telephone consultation at the start of the week with one of the other GPs who prescribed Trimethoprim for 3 days. This has not improved the symptoms and last night you had an episode of haematuria. You felt hot but have had no recorded fever, and have not had rigors or night sweats. You have not experienced any back/flank pain.

You often get 'UTI' symptoms, which you put down to not drinking enough while on shift. You have had several recent courses of antibiotics including Trimethoprim, Nitrofurantoin and Augmentin. Previous samples that have been sent to the lab have just shown 'mixed growth' and have not been very helpful.

You have no other medical problems aside from these recurrent UTIs. You think you may be going through 'the change' as you have been experiencing skin changes, hot flushes and irregular periods. You occasionally have vaginal discomfort as it feels drier and you have noticed it can be more sensitive. You are not on any medication and have no allergies.

You are married with 2 children. You rarely have intercourse with your husband, and you have had no other sexual partners.

If the candidate asks if you have taken an MSU before, say yes and explain that 'you just wee straight into the pot'.

If asked if you have any questions:

- What else could cause the bleeding?
- Could this be cancer?

## Examiner Instructions

The candidate is a Foundation Year Doctor at a GP practice. They have been asked to speak to Tamara, a 47-year-old woman who has been experiencing dysuria, frequency and abdominal pain. She has already completed a course of antibiotics for a UTI with little improvement. The candidate has been asked to take a brief, focused history and explain how to obtain a midstream urine sample. Please answer any questions she may have.

**Mark Scheme**

| Task | Achieved | Not Achieved |
|---|---|---|
| Introduces self, washes hands | | |
| Confirms name, age & occupation of patient | | |
| Establishes reason for consultation | | |
| | | |
| Asks brief history of current urinary symptoms | | |
| Takes brief medical, drug and allergy history | | |
| Asks about previous urinary symptoms, investigation and treatment | | |
| Asks about hormonal changes and associated vaginal symptoms | | |
| Establishes patients current understanding of MSU – how to take and why it is relevant | | |
| Explains why the urine sample needs to be taken mid flow | | |
| | | |
| Advises patient to wash hands before starting | | |
| Advises to use sterile bottle to store sample | | |
| Explains procedure for collecting urine sample – hold open labia, start flow, then take sample | | |
| Ensures sample has to be preserved (less than 2 hours ideally, or refrigerated if older) | | |
| Advises results usually take 48 hours | | |
| Identifies patients ideas, concerns & expectations in an empathetic manner | | |
| Discusses patients concerns about haematuria | | |
| | | |
| Summarises key points, checks understanding | | |
| Safety netting and arranges follow up | | |
| Maintains non judgemental approach | | |
| Completes station in a confident and professional manner | | |
| | | |
| Examiners Global Mark | /5 | |
| Actors Global Mark | /5 | |
| Total Station Mark | /30 | |

# Learning points

- Recurrent urinary symptoms are common in peri-menopausal women. If urine is persistently negative, consider atrophic vaginitis.

- Remember: *painless* haematuria is cancer until proven otherwise.

- As with all clinical skills – do not forget hand washing, technique, and clearing your workstation at the end – do not miss the easy marks!

# Station 20: Explaining a Hysteroscopy

## Candidate Instructions

You are the Foundation Year Doctor in the Gynaecology Clinic. Frances is a 58-year-old woman who has been experiencing postmenopausal bleeding. A transvaginal ultrasound showed a slightly thickened endometrium. She is to have an urgent hysteroscopy and you have been asked by your consultant to explain this procedure to her and discuss her concerns.

You do not need to examine the patient.

You have eight minutes.

## Actor Instructions

You are Frances, a 58-year-old writer and you have presented to the Gynaecology clinic. You have been experiencing intermittent vaginal bleeding for the past 2 months, and your GP referred you as a '2 week wait' referral to the Gynaecology team. You had an ultrasound scan last week that showed that the lining of your womb was thicker than expected, and so they have advised you to have a biopsy. You were quite upset when you found out the results of the ultrasound, as you are very afraid of it being cancer. The doctor advised you to come back in a few days to discuss the procedure to get a biopsy, which is why you are here today.

You went through the menopause over 5 years ago and have had no bleeding since you were 53 years old until now. Everything has happened quite quickly and you have not had time to process it, but the doctor advised that there are a few different options now in order to get the biopsy.

You are very anxious about having the procedure while awake and you would prefer to be asleep so you will not feel anything. You expect it is a bit like a smear test but worse, which you do find uncomfortable at the best of times.

You are otherwise well and on no medications. You have never had general anaesthetic or any surgical procedure, and you have not had any other gynaecological issues. You have no drug allergies. There is no family history of note.

Please steer the candidate away from asking a full history as you have been asked this before, and you are only here to find out about the procedure.

## Examiner Instructions

The candidate is a Foundation Year Doctor in the Gynaecology Clinic. They have been asked to speak to Frances, a 58-year-old woman who has been having postmenopausal bleeding. A transvaginal ultrasound showed a slightly thickened endometrium and she is to have an urgent hysteroscopy. They have been asked by your consultant to explain this procedure to her and discuss her concerns.

The candidate has been informed that they do not need to examine the patient.

# Mark Scheme

| Task | Achieved | Not Achieved |
|---|---|---|
| Introduces self, washes hands | | |
| Confirms name, age & occupation of patient | | |
| Establishes reason for consultation | | |
| | | |
| Takes brief history of recent symptoms and events leading up to consultation | | |
| Establishes prior knowledge of what the procedure is and why it is done | | |
| Explains causes of postmenopausal bleeding | | |
| Explains the procedure usually a day case | | |
| Can be done under general anaesthetic if preferred and a suitable candidate for this | | |
| Explains preparation before surgery | | |
| Explains what to expect during procedure and timescale | | |
| Explains what to expect after the procedure – cramping, bleeding | | |
| Advises to arrange transport home or to be with someone if under anaesthetic | | |
| Discusses recovery time | | |
| Explains procedure risks: bleeding, infection, injury to anatomy, anaesthetic risks | | |
| Advise no sexual intercourse for 7 days or until bleeding stops to reduce risk of infection | | |
| Explains will contact with results within a week | | |
| Identifies patients ideas, concerns & expectations in an empathetic manner | | |
| | | |
| Summarises key points, checks understanding & avoids jargon | | |
| Arranges follow up and offers take home info | | |
| Completes station in a confident and professional manner | | |
| | | |
| Examiners Global Mark | /5 | |
| Actors Global Mark | /5 | |
| Total Station Mark | /30 | |

## Learning points

- Separate explaining procedure stations into before, during and after the procedure to deliver more manageable 'chunks' of information. The 'chunk-and-check' approach to information delivery is effective in ensuring understanding and paced well in real life, but also in the OSCE exam to ensure you are covering all your bases (and gathering marks!).

- As is the case in this scenario, a balanced explanation should be given to the patient outlining both the benefits of the procedure but also the potential risks and complications. It may seem more stressful and difficult to describe potential complications, however informed consent cannot be given sufficient explanation of these facts.

- Hysteroscopy can be performed both in the Gynaecology outpatient department and in theatres. It can be both diagnostic and therapeutic, as most polyps and some fibroids can be removed.

# Station 21: Explaining mechanism and stages of birth

## Candidate Instructions

You are the Foundation Year Doctor in a GP surgery. Megan is a first year student midwife who has just started her community placement today. The practice midwife has just called in sick and your trainer has asked if you could talk to Megan about the mechanisms and stages of birth.

You may use the model pelvis and doll available to you.

You have eight minutes.

## Actor Instructions

You are Megan, one of the first year student midwives. Today is your first day in the community and you are meant to be shadowing the practice midwife at the GP surgery. Unfortunately, she has just called in sick and the clinic has been cancelled. The practice have kindly arranged for one of their Foundation Year doctors to give you a short talk on the mechanisms and stages of birth.

You are aware that there are three stages of labour, although you are not quite sure what happens in each stage. You have seen two births before but found it all quite emotional so cannot remember the details

The doctor will then talk you through this, and if they are using lots of jargon, ask questions to clarify.

If asked if you have any questions once they finish:

- What usually causes prolonged first stage of labour?

## Examiner Instructions

The candidate is a Foundation Year Doctor in a GP practice. They have been asked to speak to Megan, a first year student midwife who has just started her community placement today. The practice midwife has just called in sick and the candidate has been asked to talk to Megan about the mechanisms and stages of birth.

# Mark Scheme

| Task | Achieved | Not Achieved |
|---|---|---|
| Introduces self, washes hands | | |
| Confirms name and stage of training | | |
| Establishes students current knowledge base | | |
| | | |
| Identifies that there are 3 stages of labour | | |
| Explains stage 1 is split: latent & active phase | | |
| Explains latent phase is indicated by regular contractions and cervical changes | | |
| Explains active phase is from 4cm dilation onwards to full dilation (10cm) and effacement | | |
| Explains 2nd stage is from full dilation to delivery | | |
| Explains the passage of the fetus through the canal | | |
| Discusses engagement | | |
| Discusses descent and flexion | | |
| Discusses internal rotation | | |
| Discusses extension and delivery | | |
| Discusses Restitution and external rotation | | |
| Explains 3rd stage is delivery of the placenta | | |
| Uses model to clearly demonstrate stages of birth | | |
| | | |
| Summarises key points, checks understanding & avoids jargon | | |
| Asks if any further questions | | |
| Identifies causes of prolonged first stage: Power, Passage, Passenger | | |
| Completes station in a confident and professional manner | | |
| | | |
| Examiners Global Mark | /5 | |
| Actors Global Mark | /5 | |
| Total Station Mark | /30 | |

## Learning points

- It is important to inspect the station before starting and look for any aids or props that might be available to you in order to explain the process clearly – use them! It is far easier in stations like this to demonstrate with a model than to simply talk out loud and expect the listener to be able to picture it all in their head.

- This station involves time management – there are clearly definitive phases you need to cover and signposting is a useful way to inform the actor and examiner that you have taken note of the vignette.

- A pictorial record of labour (partogram) can be used once labour is established to track the initial progress of the labour. Clinicians should keep in mind that birth is a 'normal' process and should not be unnecessarily medicalised. Clinical intervention should not be offered or advised where labour is progressing normally.

# Station 22: Explaining the third stage of labour

## Candidate Instructions

You are the Foundation Year Doctor in the Obstetrics day team. The consultant today has asked if you could speak to Sarah, a medical student shadowing your team on the labour ward. She has asked you to discuss the management of the 3ʳᵈ stage of labour. Please answer any questions she may have.

You have eight minutes.

## Actor Instructions

You are Sarah, a 4th year medical student on the labour ward and you are shadowing the Obstetrics team today. One of the Foundation Year Doctors has been asked to speak to you today about the management of the third stage of labour.

At present, you are aware that the 3rd stage involved the delivery of the placenta. You have seen some births on the unit and seen the midwives give that mother an injection when the baby is delivered but you are not sure what this is. You are aware that the 3rd stage can be actively or passively managed but not quite sure how these are different.

If the candidate does do not address the following, please ask these questions:

- What is the difference between active and passive management of the 3rd stage?
- What does the oxytocin do?
- How long should the first stage of labour last if oxytocin is given? How long would the 3rd stage of labour last if not?
- How do you remove the placenta?
- What causes major bleeding after giving birth?

## Examiner Instructions

The candidate is the Foundation Year Doctor in the Obstetrics day team. The consultant today has asked if they could speak to Sarah, a medical student shadowing your team on the labour ward. She would like to discuss the management of the 3$^{rd}$ stage of labour. The candidate should answer any questions she may have.

# Mark Scheme

| Task | Achieved | Not Achieved |
|---|---|---|
| Introduces self, washes hands | | |
| Confirms name and stage of training | | |
| Establishes students current knowledge base and aim of discussion | | |
| | | |
| Defines the 3$^{rd}$ stage of labour | | |
| Discusses options of active and passive (physiological) management | | |
| Discusses the difference in duration of 3$^{rd}$ stage with active and passive management | | |
| Explains passive management of cord – not clamped until pulsation stopped | | |
| Explains passive delivery of placenta with maternal effort only once naturally detaches | | |
| Explains increased risk of maternal PPH and transfusion with passive management | | |
| Explains active management involves the use of syntometrine (uterotonic drugs) | | |
| Discusses deferred clamping & cutting of cord (unless concerns about fetus or cord integrity) | | |
| Explains controlled cord traction once evidence of placental separation | | |
| Explains signs of placental separation | | |
| Explains the need to inspect the placenta to check complete and appears healthy | | |
| Explains how to manage retained placenta | | |
| Explains importance of monitoring mother for signs of blood loss | | |
| States causes of primary PPH (4 'T's) | | |
| | | |
| Summarises key points, checks understanding | | |
| Asks if any further questions | | |
| Completes station in a confident and professional manner | | |
| | | |
| Examiners Global Mark | /5 | |
| Actors Global Mark | /5 | |
| Total Station Mark | /30 | |

## Learning points

- Active management of the 3rd stage of delivery with synthetic oxytocin has a reduced rate of post-partum haemorrhage and serious complications compared to non-active management. A woman who is deemed to be low risk for postpartum haemorrhage and who requests physiological management, should of course have her request respected.

- The anatomy of the uterine muscle fibres help with haemostasis - the 'criss-cross' structure constricts blood vessels when they contract.

- During passive management, the umbilical cord is not clamped until pulsation has stopped completely. In active management, the cord is clamped 1-5 minutes after the birth and cut soon after the delivery. Delayed clamping is recommended as it can improve haemoglobin levels and reduce the risk of iron deficiency in the baby (*NICE, Sept 2016*).

# Examinations

## Station 23: Cervical Smear & Bimanual exam

### Candidate Instructions

You are the Foundation Year Doctor in a GP surgery. Sia is 25-year-old woman who has presented with PV discharge and intermittent bleeding. You have been asked to perform a cervical smear and bimanual examination. She has already been consented for the procedure.

Please use the model provided.

You have eight minutes.

## Actor Instructions

Your name is Sia and you are a 25-year-old PR manager. You have come in to the GP surgery today to have a vaginal examination and cervical smear. You have already consented to have the procedure and understand the risks and benefits.

Decline a chaperone if offered.

The candidate will perform a bimanual examination and cervical smear on a mannequin but should communicate with you as though you are being examined.

# Examiner Instructions

The candidate is a Foundation Year Doctor in a GP surgery. Sia is 25-year-old woman who has presented with PV discharge and intermittent bleeding. They have been asked to perform a cervical smear and bimanual examination. The patient has already been consented for the procedure.

## Mark Scheme

| Task | Achieved | Not Achieved |
|---|---|---|
| Introduces self, washes hands | | |
| Confirms name, age & occupation | | |
| Establishes purpose of consultation and seeks permission | | |
| Requests chaperone, asks if patient prefers door locked | | |
| Expose and Reposition patient | | |
| Prepares equipment: cytobrush, lubricating gel, speculum (checks speculum and screw) | | |
| | | |
| Inspect vulva and mentions appearance or abnormalities seen | | |
| Part labia and insert speculum using correct technique | | |
| Inspect cervix for abnormalities | | |
| Insert cytobrush into external os and rotate 360 degree 3 times | | |
| Break off head of brush into specimen pot | | |
| Unscrew and remove speculum, cover patient | | |
| Label and date specimen pots | | |
| Perform bimanual exam – two gloved & lubricated fingers close to posterior fornix | | |
| Applies pressure to suprapubic area, comments on uterus, palpates adnexae | | |
| Covers and thanks patient, clears workspace | | |
| | | |
| Safety netting, discusses results and follow up | | |
| Summarises key points, checks understanding | | |
| Asks if any further questions | | |
| Completes station in a confident and professional manner | | |
| | | |
| Examiners Global Mark | /5 | |
| Actors Global Mark | /5 | |
| Total Station Mark | /30 | |

## Learning points

- In examination stations, remember to address the actor as the actual patient, as communication skills are still assessed. Most patients will appreciate you talking through what you are doing in real time both to prepare them for what is coming, but also to explain the reasons for why you are doing the various parts of the examination.

- Always request a chaperone for any intimate examinations and ensure that their details are documented in the notes. Having another person present can ensure both the patient and doctor feel supported.

- The bimanual examination is able to assess for abnormalities in the vaginal vault, to palpate the cervix for lumps or excitation, to assess the uterine position, size and tenderness and to examine the adnexae for swellings or tenderness.

# Station 24:
# Examination of the Pregnant Abdomen

## Candidate Instructions

You are the Foundation Year Doctor in the General Obstetrics clinic. Lucy is 28-year-old woman who is currently 28 weeks pregnant. She has come in for a routine check. You have been asked to perform an examination of her pregnant abdomen. Please present your findings to the examiner and discuss.

Please use the mannequin provided.

You have eight minutes.

## Actor Instructions

Your name is Lucy and you are a 28-year-old fashion editor. You have come in to the General Obstetrics Clinic today for a routine check up at 28 weeks as you have been diagnosed with Gestational Diabetes (only give this information if asked). You feel well and have had no pain and your sugars are well controlled.

The candidate has been asked to examine your pregnant abdomen (for which they will use the mannequin provided). They should, however, communicate with you as though you are being examined.

If the candidate does not ask if you are in any pain before examining, please express your discomfort.

## Examiner Instructions

The candidate is a Foundation Year Doctor in the General Obstetrics clinic. They have been asked to examine the pregnant abdomen of a 28-year-old woman, Lucy, who is currently 28 weeks pregnant. She has come in for a routine check.

The candidate should then present their findings to you and please ask the following questions:

- The fundal height is 32cm. Is this normal or abnormal?
- Please give examples of what may cause this measurement.

**Mark Scheme**

| Task | Achieved | Not Achieved |
|---|---|---|
| Introduces self, washes hands | | |
| Confirms name, age & occupation | | |
| Establishes purpose of consultation and seeks permission | | |
| Exposes and repositions patient | | |
| Asks if in any pain or discomfort | | |
| | | |
| Inspects abdomen for scars, striae & linea nigra | | |
| Assesses fundal height – informs patient this may be uncomfortable | | |
| Palpate contents or abdomen to locate head, back and limbs | | |
| Comment on lie i.e.: transverse, longitudinal | | |
| Comment on presentation (i.e. breech, cephalic) | | |
| Determine position of head in pelvis (occiput in relation to anterior pelvis – i.e. LOA, ROA) | | |
| Determine how many fifths palpable above pelvic brim | | |
| Comments on liquor volume | | |
| Offers to assess fetal heartbeat | | |
| Covers & thanks the patient, clears workspace | | |
| Comments on further assessments to complete exam (BP, peripheral oedema, urine dipstick) | | |
| | | |
| Summarises findings in clear and concise manner | | |
| Identifies larger than expected fundal height | | |
| Able to give causes of polyhydramnios | | |
| Completes station in a confident and professional manner | | |
| | | |
| Examiners Global Mark | /5 | |
| Actors Global Mark | /5 | |
| Total Station Mark | /30 | |

## Learning points

- Assessing the fetal lie is something that comes with practice. By applying gentle but sustained pressure to either side of the uterus, one side should appear fuller indicating the fetal back is there, and the opposite side may allow you to palpate fetal limbs. The lie may be described as longitudinal, transverse or oblique.

- Know the causes of polyhydramnios and oligohydramnios – fundal height from pubic symphysis to fundus in centimetres (+/-2cm) should correlate with the number of weeks gestation up till 20 weeks at least.

- Examination of the fetal heart is often the most anticipated and stressful part of the examination for both patient and doctor. Use of a hand held Doppler or Pinard stethosope is essential and the fetal heart rate should be between 110-160bpm. Comparison with the mother's radial pulse can ensure you are happy it is indeed that of the fetus.

# Counselling Stations

## Station 25: Discussing Cervical Smear Results

### Candidate Instructions

You are the Foundation Year Doctor in a GP surgery. Gina is a 35-year-old woman who has been sent a letter asking to attend a routine appointment at her GP surgery due to abnormal smear results. You have the results that states:

Mild dyskaryosis, HPV positive.

Please counsel the patient regarding investigation and follow up in view of these findings and answer any questions she may have.

You do not need to examine the patient.

You have eight minutes.

## Actor Instructions

You are Gina, a 35-year-old fashion editor. You have received a letter from your GP to come into the surgery to discuss the results from your recent smear. You are worried because you have not received such a letter before. All previous smears have shown no abnormalities.

You are otherwise fit and well and have had no symptoms. You are married with 2 young girls aged 2 and 4.

You searched online about what an abnormality could mean and have questions related to changes that could be present. You are worried that this means you have cancer, and you don't know how you would cope with such a diagnosis.

If asked for questions and not already covered:
- What is HPV?
- What does CIN mean?
- What happens when I go for colposcopy?
- What have I done to get this and is there anything that I can do to prevent it?
- Is there anything I can do to reduce my risk of getting this?
- Is it hereditary? Will my daughters be at risk?

# Examiner Instructions

The candidate is a Foundation Year Doctor based at a GP practice. Gina is a 35-year-old woman who has been sent a letter asking to attend a routine appointment at her GP surgery due to abnormal smear results. The results state:

Mild dyskaryosis, HPV positive.

They have been asked to counsel the patient in view of these findings and answer any questions she may have. They do not need to examine the patient.

## Mark Scheme

| Task | Achieved | Not Achieved |
|---|---|---|
| Introduces self, washes hands | | |
| Confirms name, age & occupation of patient | | |
| Establishes reason for consultation | | |
| | | |
| Discusses previous smear results or symptoms | | |
| Establishes patient's current knowledge of cervical smear outcomes | | |
| Explains CIN is cervical intraepithelial neoplasm and describes changes in the cervical squamous cells | | |
| Sensitively explains 'mild dyskaryosis' and HPV positive | | |
| Explains that changes in cells seen on smear could indicate CIN | | |
| Reassures patient that CIN is NOT cancer | | |
| Discusses that CIN I can progress to II or III | | |
| Explains if CIN II or III are untreated, it can progress to cervical cancer | | |
| Explains HPV is sexually transmitted | | |
| Explains it is usually asymptomatic but certain types can increase risk of warts or cancer | | |
| Explains plan to refer for routine colposcopy | | |
| Explains colposcopy investigation, can take biopsy and treat if required | | |
| Explains not hereditary, but vaccination given to 12-year-olds to prevent certain strains of HPV | | |
| | | |
| Identifies patient's ideas, concerns and expectations in an empathetic manner | | |
| Summarises key points, checks understanding & avoids jargon | | |
| Suggests follow up or take home information | | |
| Completes station in a confident and professional manner | | |
| | | |
| Examiners Global Mark | /5 | |
| Actors Global Mark | /5 | |
| Total Station Mark | /30 | |

# Learning points

- Ensure the patient understands this is NOT a diagnosis of cancer, and be able to clearly explain the risks associated with untreated CIN. Approximately a third of women with CIN II or III will go on to develop cancer over the next 10 years. CIN I is less concerning as it commonly regresses, but can also progress to CIN II or III.

- Learn about all possible outcomes of a cervical smear: negative, borderline, mild, moderate or severe dyskaryosis and relevant further investigation.

- Understand how cervical cancer develops and pathophysiology including in relation to HPV. HPV inactivates important tumour suppressor genes and this, in conjuction with other mutations, can lead to cancer.

# Station 26: Oral Contraceptive Pill

## Candidate Instructions

You are the Foundation Year Doctor in a GP surgery. Celia is an 18-year-old woman who has asked to speak to you about starting the oral contraceptive pill. Please counsel the patient regarding the oral contraceptive pill and answer any questions she may have. Please also ask a focused history to elicit suitability for the chosen method of contraception.

You do not need to examine the patient.

You have eight minutes.

## Actor Instructions

You are Celia, an 18-year-old university student. You have asked to speak to your GP today as you are thinking about starting the oral contraceptive pill.

You have been with your boyfriend for the past 6 months and have been sexually active for the last 4 months. Your boyfriend is 20 years old. You have only been using condoms until now, but you want to explore other forms of contraception. You spoke to your friends who suggested the 'combined' contraceptive pill. You are keen to start the combined pill, but you also wanted to know a little more about the progesterone-only pill as well.

Your boyfriend is your only current sexual partner. You have never had an STI, and your partner had a negative STI check prior to starting sexual intercourse. You have not noticed any vaginal discharge. Your menstrual cycle is regular occurring every 28 days and lasting for 5 days. You do not have very heavy menstruation or irregular bleeding. You have never been pregnant.

Your only significant past medical history includes mild asthma for which you use a salbutamol inhaler as required. You have no history of migraines. You have no other regular medications or allergies. You smoke 5 cigarettes a day. You do not regularly drink during the week, but may have 2-3 glasses of wine on a night out over the weekend. You are not overweight.

Your family history includes a mother who is hypertensive and a father who is diabetic and a smoker.

You have some specific questions about the use of the combined oral contraceptive pill:
- What are you chances of getting pregnant while on the COCP?
- What are the side effects?
- Can you still contract a STI?
- Is there an increasing risk of getting cancer?
- What happens if I miss a pill?
- Will the pill affect my long-term fertility once I come off of it?

## Examiner Instructions

The candidate is a Foundation Year Doctor based at a GP practice. Celia is an 18-year-old woman who has asked to talk about starting the oral contraceptive pill. The candidate has been asked to counsel the patient regarding the oral contraceptive pill and answer any questions she may have. They have been asked to take a focused history to elicit suitability for the chosen method of contraception. They do not need to examine the patient.

**Mark Scheme**

| Task | Achieved | Not Achieved |
|---|---|---|
| Introduces self, washes hands | | |
| Confirms name, age & occupation of patient | | |
| Establishes reason for consultation | | |
| | | |
| Establishes patient's current knowledge of oral contraceptive methods | | |
| Discusses 2 types of OCP – COCP or POP | | |
| Explains the mechanism of the COCP | | |
| Discusses advantages of COCP and efficacy (perfect and typical use) | | |
| Discusses disadvantages of COCP – compliance, common side effects, risk of STIs | | |
| Discusses differences and benefits of POP | | |
| Takes focused history to elicit suitability for COCP, directly asking about contraindications | | |
| Able to identify she is suitable for COCP | | |
| Discusses initiating pill, also mentioning need for additional cover if starting after day 5 of cycle | | |
| Discusses increased and reduced risks of different forms of cancer | | |
| Discusses missed pill management | | |
| Discuss need for caution with over the counter/prescription meds | | |
| Informs patient long term fertility unaffected | | |
| | | |
| Identifies patient's ideas, concerns and expectations in an empathetic manner | | |
| Summarises key points, checks understanding & avoids jargon | | |
| Suggests follow up or take home information | | |
| Completes station in a confident and professional manner | | |
| | | |
| Examiners Global Mark | /5 | |
| Actors Global Mark | /5 | |
| Total Station Mark | /30 | |

# Learning points

- Remember – the oral contraceptive pill slightly increases the risk of breast and cervical cancer but reduces the risk of ovarian, endometrial and bowel cancer.

- Missed pill information is very easy to get confused about for patients. If the patient forgets to take a progestogen-only pill (POP), they must take it as soon as they remember. It is important to remind the patient that if they are more than three hours late in taking it (or more than 12 hours with a third generation POP) then the protection immediately fails. They must continue to take the POP each day, but will need to use extra contraception (such as condoms) for two more days before the POP becomes effective again.

- VTE risk is notably higher in women on the COCP (2 per 10 000 women in general population, 5-12 per 10 000 in combined hormonal contraception users (*FSRH, 2014*)). It is true however that for most women the overall benefits outweigh the overall risks. Each woman should be risk assessed and then stratified for suitability.

# Station 27: Long-acting Contraceptive Therapy

## Candidate Instructions

You are the Foundation Year Doctor in a GP surgery. Tiana is a 25-year-old woman who has come to see her GP. She would like to discuss switching to a long-acting contraceptive and would like some more information about what is available. Please counsel her on the available options take a focused history to elicit her suitability for her chosen method.

You do not need to examine the patient.

You have eight minutes.

## Actor Instructions

You are Tiana, a 25-year-old fitness instructor. You have presented to the GP surgery as you want to discuss a more long-term contraceptive method. You would like to know more about the available options.

You recently got married and you have been using the contraceptive pill for the past 5 years. You have struggled with your skin and weight changes and have switched pills a few times over the years. You are interested in trying a more long-term method as you and your husband wanted to wait a few years before starting a family. You have been reading up about the coil but you were not sure if the copper or hormone coil would be best. If all options are discussed, please inform the candidate you would like to talk more about the intrauterine options.

Your husband is your only current sexual partner. You have never had an STI. Your last STI screen was over 2 years ago prior to starting sexual intercourse with your husband. You have not noticed any vaginal discharge. You have never been pregnant. You take the COCP and have your menstrual cycle every 21 days. Prior to this you had heavy, painful periods. Your last smear test was 4 months ago and was normal. You are not known to have any structural problems with your womb.

You have no significant past medical history and exercise regularly – your BMI is 23. You do not have any allergies, and do not take any regular medication apart from the OCP. You do not smoke. You drink 6-7 units of alcohol a week. Your family history includes a father who is hypertensive and diabetic.

You have some specific questions about the intrauterine system:
1. How long after stopping will I be able to conceive?
2. What are the side effects?
3. How will it affect my periods

At the end of the consultation, you would like to go away and think about your options before making a decision.

## Examiner Instructions

The candidate is a Foundation Year Doctor in a GP surgery. Tiana is a 25-year-old woman who has come to see her GP. She would like to discuss switching to a long-acting contraceptive and would like some more information about what is available. They have been asked to counsel her on contraceptive options and take a focused history to elicit her suitability.

They do not need to examine the patient.

**Mark Scheme**

| Task | Achieved | Not Achieved |
|---|---|---|
| Introduces self, washes hands | | |
| Confirms name, age & occupation of patient | | |
| Establishes reason for consultation | | |
| | | |
| Establishes patient's current knowledge of available options | | |
| Discusses overall benefit of LARC (not user dependent) but no STI protection | | |
| Discusses 4 types of LARC – IUD, IUS, implant and depot injection | | |
| Explains the mechanism of the IUS and IUD | | |
| Explains mechanism of implant | | |
| Explains mechanism of the depot injection | | |
| Discusses advantages of coil and efficacy | | |
| Discusses disadvantages of IUS | | |
| Discusses important risks of insertion – perforation, dislodged device, ectopic, PID | | |
| Discusses advantages and disadvantages of IUD – mentions heavy menstruation | | |
| Able to recommend IUS over IUD based on the history of heavy painful periods | | |
| Takes focused history to elicit suitability for IUS, directly asking about contraindications | | |
| Informs patient long term fertility is not affected by the coil | | |
| | | |
| Identifies patient's ideas, concerns and expectations in an empathetic manner | | |
| Summarises key points, checks understanding & avoids jargon | | |
| Suggests follow up or take home information | | |
| Completes station in a confident and professional manner | | |
| | | |
| Examiners Global Mark | /5 | |
| Actors Global Mark | /5 | |
| Total Station Mark | /30 | |

## Learning points

- Long acting reversible contraception (LARC) is NOT protective against STIs – make sure you inform patients barrier protection is the only form of protection that reduces the transmission of STIs.

- If the IUS is inserted within the first 7 days of the cycle, no additional contraception is required. However, after this, an additional form of contraception is required for 7 days. The IUS can remain in place for 3-5 years, depending on the type. The copper IUD can be inserted at any point in the cycle (if certain that the patient is not pregnant), and can remain in situ for 5-10 years, depending on the type. Fertility returns to normal as soon as either device is removed.

- The IUS acts by thinning the endometrium, thickening cervical mucus and may also stop ovulation. The IUD is a copper, non-hormonal coil that acts by preventing sperm from surviving to reach the egg and by stopping implantation. Both are 99% effective and not user dependent.

# Station 28: Hormone Replacement Therapy

## Candidate Instructions

You are the Foundation Year Doctor in a GP surgery. Florence is a 49-year-old woman who has recently been experiencing hot flushes and has stopped having periods for 10 months. She would like to discuss starting hormone replacement therapy.

Please counsel her on available options of HRT and take a focused history to elicit her suitability, answering any questions she may have.

You do not need to examine the patient.

You have ten minutes.

## Actor Instructions

You are Florence, a 49-year-old teacher. You have presented to the GP today as you have been experiencing hot flushes and have had no periods for 10 months. You have put this down to approaching the menopause. You have heard about hormone replacement therapy from your friends and would like to know more information about starting it.

Your last proper period was about 10 months ago, but for the first few months you had some irregular, light bleeds which may have been around the time you would expect your period. You have noticed you experience more frequent hot flushes, and often find it hard to sleep at night. You have noticed vaginal dryness, which has made intercourse with your husband uncomfortable. You have also noticed your skin appears tired and dry.

You started your menstrual cycle at the age of 13. Your normal cycle is normally every 28 days lasting for 5 days. You have never had problems with irregular or heavy bleeding. You have had 2 normal vaginal deliveries. You have never had an STI. You are infrequently sexually active with your husband. You have not had a hysterectomy.

Your have no medical problems or medications and no allergies. You have never had a fall or any fractures. You do not have a history of breast cancer, heart disease or a history of clots. You do not drink alcohol or smoke. Your family history includes a mother who passed away following a stroke aged 65 years.

You are worried you may have started the menopause early. You are distressed by some of your symptoms, and after speaking to your friends, you are worried that it may go on for years. As a result, you would like to know more about HRT. You have some specific questions:

1. I have heard it can stop the hot flushes. What other benefits are there?
2. Do I need to take it every day?
3. Do I continue to take it forever?
4. Does this mean I do not need to use contraception or is there something that can do both?
5. What would be the most suitable type of HRT for me?

## Examiner Instructions

The candidate is a Foundation Year Doctor based at a GP practice. Florence is a 49-year-old woman who has recently been experiencing hot flushes and has stopped having regular periods for 10 months. She would like to discuss hormone replacement therapy.

They have been asked to counsel her on available options of HRT and take a focused history to elicit her suitability, answering any questions she may have.

**Mark Scheme**

| Task | Achieved | Not Achieved |
|---|---|---|
| Introduces self, washes hands | | |
| Confirms name, age & occupation of patient | | |
| Establishes reason for consultation | | |
| | | |
| Establishes patient's current knowledge of HRT | | |
| Takes history of current perimenopausal symptoms: e.g. skin, hot flushes, dryness, mood | | |
| Asks brief gynaecological and obstetric history | | |
| Takes focused medical, drug, family and social history to elicit suitability | | |
| Checks if patient has had hysterectomy | | |
| Discusses advantages of HRT | | |
| Discusses disadvantages HRT | | |
| Highlights contraindications for taking HRT | | |
| Discusses different types of HRT available | | |
| Specifies that it cannot be used as sole form of contraception during perimenopausal period | | |
| Discusses duration of therapy | | |
| Advises sequential/cyclic therapy is suitable as she has had periods in the last 12 months | | |
| Advises IUS with oral/patch oestrogen can serve as both HRT and contraception | | |
| | | |
| Identifies patient's ideas, concerns and expectations in an empathetic manner | | |
| Summarises key points, checks understanding & avoids jargon | | |
| Suggests follow up or take home information | | |
| Completes station in a confident and professional manner | | |
| | | |
| Examiners Global Mark | /5 | |
| Actors Global Mark | /5 | |
| Total Station Mark | /30 | |

## Learning points

- It is important to remember that women who have a uterus should NOT be given unopposed oestrogen as this can increase the risk of endometrial cancer.

- HRT can reduce the risk of osteoporosis and fractures, as well as colorectal cancer. If early natural or surgical menopause (onset before 45 years), patients should be given HRT until the natural age of menopause (i.e. 50 years) due to the high risk of developing osteoporosis (*BNF, 2016*).

- The British National Formulary (BNF) recommends that the minimum dose of HRT should be given for the minimum length of time, and use should be reviewed annually at least. If HRT is solely being prescribed for the prevention of osteoporosis, an alternative should be used (*BNF, 2016*).

# Station 29: HIV Pre-test Counselling

## Candidate Instructions

You are the Foundation Year Doctor in the Genitourinary Medicine (GUM) clinic. Marc is a 19-year-old man who has come in for a routine STI screen after having had unprotected sexual intercourse with a casual partner. Please take a focused history and counsel this patient for a HIV test. You do not need to examine the patient.

You have ten minutes.

## Actor Instructions

You are Marc, a 19-year-old choreographer. You have presented to the GUM clinic today after having unprotected sexual intercourse with a casual partner last week and wanted a routine STI check.

You are bisexual, but in the last 6 months, you have had 3 male partners. You are usually very careful with using condoms, but on this one occasion you were quite drunk and got carried away in the moment. You are concerned that you could have contracted HIV. You are currently only sleeping with this one casual partner for the last 3 months, prior to which you had a negative HIV and STI check, but you do not know about your partner. On this occasion, you had anal, oral and oro-anal sex – both reciprocal and penetrative.

You have not travelled abroad to any high-risk areas. You have not had any previous partners with known HIV or from high-risk areas. You have never used intravenous drugs and have never had any blood transfusions and you do not believe your partner has either. You have never paid anyone for sex.

You currently feel well with no penile or anal symptoms. About a week ago you had a flu-like illness but that has now settled. You have no other medical history aside from treated chlamydia 3 years ago.

If asked, you would like to know:

- How the test will be taken
- How long will I have to wait before the results come back and how will they be given
- What is HIV? How is it transmitted? Is there treatment for it?
- Are there any other ways to protect myself from contracting HIV?

If the HIV test returned with a positive result, you would be devastated. You have heard it is a 'death sentence' and you are scared that it would change all your future life plans. You would be worried about being able to have a long-term relationship if you had HIV. You have a very supportive family and so you have a good support network to help you if the test came back positive.

## Examiner Instructions

The candidate is a Foundation Year Doctor in the GUM clinic. Marc is a 19-year-old man who has come in for a routine STI screen after having had unprotected sexual intercourse with a casual partner. They have been asked to take a focused history and counsel this patient for a HIV test, but they do not need to examine the patient.

**Mark Scheme**

| Task | Achieved | Not Achieved |
|------|----------|--------------|
| Introduces self, washes hands | | |
| Confirms name, age & occupation of patient | | |
| Establishes reason for consultation and identifies why they want to be tested | | |
| | | |
| Gives warning shot re sensitive questions and reiterates confidentiality | | |
| Asks about sexual partners in last 6 months: gender, type of sex and contraceptive use | | |
| Asks about high risk behaviour for HIV/Hepatitis e.g. IVDU, travel, background of partner | | |
| Asks about previous and current STIs and completion of treatment | | |
| | | |
| Checks current level of understanding about HIV and knowledge of transmission risk | | |
| Explains what HIV is | | |
| Explains the test procedure | | |
| Explains test limitation (3 month window period) | | |
| Identifies implications of having a positive or negative test result | | |
| Explains how long until results come back and how they will be communicated | | |
| Checks how patient would cope with positive result, asks about support network | | |
| Asks patient if still happy to have the test | | |
| | | |
| Identifies patient's ideas, concerns and expectations in an empathetic manner | | |
| Summarises key points, checks understanding & avoids jargon | | |
| Suggests follow up or take home information | | |
| Completes station in a confident and professional manner | | |
| | | |
| Examiners Global Mark | /5 | |
| Actors Global Mark | /5 | |
| Total Station Mark | /30 | |

# Learning points

- Pre-exposure prophylaxis (PrEP) has been shown to be very effective in reducing the transmission of disease in high-risk individuals. This can either be taken daily if consistently at risk, or 'on-demand' before and after sex. Currently, this is not available on the NHS but can be purchased privately. It does not protect against other STIs or the risk of pregnancy.

- Patients will need to be retested If exposure was within the last 3 months as there is a window period where a patient may test negative and the virus may not be detectable.

- Ask about any recent non-specific symptoms that could represent a seroconversion illness. This usually occurs 1 to 4 weeks following exposure and is noted to be a 'flu-like' illness with non-specific symptoms. This includes lethargy, fever, rash, lymphadenopathy, and muscle/joint pains.

# Station 30: New Diagnosis of HIV

## Candidate Instructions

You are the Foundation Year Doctor in the Genitourinary Medicine (GUM) clinic. David is a 27-year-old man who was diagnosed with HIV in a routine STI check and informed last week at the clinic. He has come back today for follow up. Please answer any questions he may have, but you do not need to examine the patient.

You have ten minutes.

## Actor Instructions

You are David, a 27-year-old photographer. You have come back to the GUM clinic today to discuss your new diagnosis of HIV last week. You have been quite shell-shocked, as it was totally unexpected. You have not yet told your family but you told one of your oldest friends who has been reassuring and helpful to talk to.

Today you have written down a few questions about how this happened and what happens now.

You are otherwise well with no other medical, drug or family history. You have been sexually active since you were 15 years old and only ever in a heterosexual relationship. You have never done drugs and do not smoke. You drink only at the weekend, and tend to binge drink when out with friends.

Three months ago you went to Malia on a boy's holiday and had a few episodes of unprotected sex with 3 or 4 unfamiliar partners. You are currently not in a relationship.

You are quite concerned about informing your manager as they have made lots of cuts to staff because of 'budget cuts'. You are worried that they will use this as an excuse to fire you, because people might be scared that they may catch it.

Questions you would like to ask:

- How long do I have to live?
- Is it the same as AIDS?
- Can I still have sex?
- If so, can I still have children?
- Do I need to tell my workplace occupational health team?
- When do I need to start treatment?
- How do I know if the disease is getting worse?

## Examiner Instructions

The candidate is a Foundation Year Doctor in the GUM clinic. David is a 27-year-old man who was diagnosed with HIV in a routine STI check and informed last week at the clinic. He has come back today for follow up. The candidate has been asked to answer any questions he may have, but they do not need to examine the patient.

**Mark Scheme**

| Task | Achieved | Not Achieved |
|---|---|---|
| Introduces self, washes hands | | |
| Confirms name, age & occupation of patient | | |
| Establishes reason for consultation | | |
| | | |
| Establish what the patient remembers from the last meeting | | |
| Ask how patient has been coping and what support they have | | |
| Allows patient to lead discussion with questions | | |
| Reassures patient that many patients have a normal lifespan with follow up and treatment | | |
| Discusses the difference between HIV and AIDS | | |
| Reassures patient that they can continue to have sexual intercourse with barrier protection | | |
| Reassures patient that he can still have children and discusses options for doing so safely | | |
| Discusses transmission methods and how to reduce risks | | |
| Reassures about confidentiality, no need to inform workplace if irrelevant to job description | | |
| Explores concerns about informing workplace | | |
| Reiterates confidentiality in clinical session, within the parameters set by GMC | | |
| Discusses general treatment options | | |
| Explains monitoring viral load and CD4 count | | |
| | | |
| Identifies patient's ideas, concerns and expectations in an empathetic manner | | |
| Summarises key points, checks understanding & avoids jargon | | |
| Suggests follow up or take home information | | |
| Completes station in a confident and professional manner | | |
| | | |
| Examiners Global Mark | /5 | |
| Actors Global Mark | /5 | |
| Total Station Mark | /30 | |

## Learning points

- You do not need to have extensive knowledge about specialist medications for the treatment of HIV, but an understanding of the mechanisms of action with 1-2 examples will help in this scenario and also in the written exam.

- It is important to clarify what the patient can remember from their last meeting. When breaking bad news, patients rarely retain much information due to the shock of the diagnosis. Always check what needs to be covered again to make sure the patient is fully informed.

- When counselling a patient, it is important to consider psychosocial issues in the OSCE and in real life. Explore their support network and concerns regarding the cultural and social stigma that still surrounds HIV. Confidentiality with friends, work colleagues and their other medical should be stressed. This diagnosis is not one that needs to be shared widely without the patient's consent.

# Station 31: Needlestick Injury from HIV patient

## Candidate Instructions

You are the Foundation Year Doctor in the Emergency Department. Tinashe is a 23-year-old final year medical student who has booked in after a needlestick injury whilst taking blood from a HIV-positive patient on the ward.

Please take a focused history from her and discuss management.

You do not need to examine the patient.

You have eight minutes.

## Actor Instructions

You are Tinashe, a 23-year-old final year medical student. You have presented to the Emergency Department after sustaining a needlestick injury while taking blood from a HIV-positive patient on the Respiratory Ward half an hour ago. The nursing staff advised you to come to ED for further assessment. You are very worried that you may have contracted HIV from the injury.

You were wearing gloves at the time but the needle did go through the glove and puncture the skin. This happened after successfully taking venous blood from the patient. The injury happened as you went to dispose of the needle in the sharps bin, then fumbled and pricked yourself. You squeezed and washed the area for a few minutes under the running tap.

You know the patient is HIV positive but do not know his recent viral load or CD4 count, but he had presented with breathlessness and was admitted with Pneumocystis Pneumonia. You are not sure of his hepatitis B or C status. You had routine checks for HIV and Hepatitis B and C when you started medical school but have not been checked since.

If asked, you would like to know:
- What is the risk of contracting HIV from this injury?
- Do I need to start any treatment at this point?
- What are the main side effects of treatment?
- Do any further tests need to be done?
- How will this impact my clinical experience?

You are anxious about the implications that a positive HIV test result would have, both personally and professionally.

## Examiner Instructions

The candidate is a Foundation Year Doctor in the Emergency Department. Tinashe is a 23-year-old final year medical student who has booked in after a needlestick injury whilst taking blood from a HIV-positive patient on the ward. They have been asked to take a focused history from her and discuss management.

They do not need to examine the patient.

## Mark Scheme

| Task | Achieved | Not Achieved |
|---|---|---|
| Introduces self, washes hands | | |
| Confirms name, age & stage of training | | |
| Establishes reason for consultation | | |
| | | |
| Checks how long since the injury occurred | | |
| Asks if gloves were worn and if the needle had punctured the skin | | |
| Asks if injury occurred before or after taking blood from patient, and if flashback was noted | | |
| Asks if puncture site was squeezed and washed | | |
| Asks about donor's HIV status and if infectivity known (i.e. CD4/viral load) | | |
| Explains that patient will need to be consented and bled by other healthcare staff | | |
| Advises to contact Occupational Health | | |
| Advises to complete Datix/incident report | | |
| Discusses transmission rate of HIV and Hep B/C | | |
| Explains need for post exposure prophylaxis and associated side effects | | |
| Advises regarding repeat blood tests to check viral serology and monitor for effects of PEP | | |
| Discusses precautions until HIV status known – safe sex, no blood donation for 3-6 months | | |
| Discusses refraining from clinical duties with risk of blood borne virus transmission | | |
| | | |
| Identifies patient's ideas, concerns and expectations in an empathetic manner | | |
| Summarises key points, checks understanding & avoids jargon | | |
| Suggests follow up or take home information | | |
| Completes station in a confident and professional manner | | |
| | | |
| Examiners Global Mark | /5 | |
| Actors Global Mark | /5 | |
| Total Station Mark | /30 | |

# Learning points

- Demonstrating empathy and sensitivity is key in a scenario like this, which you can understand would be nerve-racking in real life. The global marks from the actor and examiner will reflect your ability to manage the situation appropriately. Giving the patient time to share their concerns is essential - do not rush them.

- Know details of PEP and it's side effects and advice for student regarding clinical practice. Health care professionals will require follow up in occupational health to make them aware of what clinical areas may not be suitable until a definitive answer is available on the risk and transmission.

- Stations could be altered to counselling for a needlestick injury from a patient with Hepatitis B or C instead of HIV. Make sure you learn the transmission rates and advice for Hepatitis as well as HIV (*CDC, 2003*).

  0.3% for percutaneous exposure to HIV-infected blood
  0.1% for mucocutaneous exposure to HIV-infected blood.
  0.5-1.8% for percutaneous exposure to HCV-infected blood with detectable RNA.
  30% for percutaneous exposure of a non-immune individual to an HBeAg positive source

# Station 32: Chlamydia Contact Tracing

## Candidate Instructions

You are the Foundation Year Doctor in the Genitourinary Medicine (GUM) clinic. Frank is a 19-year-old man who has presented after receiving a text telling him that he's been in contact with someone who has Chlamydia. Please take a focused history and counsel him about how this will be managed. You do not need to examine the patient.

You have eight minutes.

## Actor Instructions

You are Frank, a 19-year-old man in your first year of university. You have presented to the GUM clinic today after receiving a text saying you have been in contact with someone with Chlamydia. The candidate has been asked to speak to you about what this means and take a brief history from you.

You are single and have had 7 male sexual partners in the last 3 months. At first you were careful to use condoms, but at times you were quite drunk and cannot always remember wearing one.

You are usually 'on top' (penetrating) but have tried being 'on the bottom' (reciprocator) with your last partner, and you do not know if he wore a condom. You once paid for sex (with a man) and you both wore a condom. You don't inject drugs nor have had sex with anyone from HIV/hepatitis prevalent areas. You've never had a blood transfusion.

You have no pain, dysuria or abnormal discharge. You have no other medical problems and currently feel well.

You'd like to know what this text message means. As you've had no symptoms, you don't understand how you could have chlamydia. You are also concerned you could have other diseases without knowing, especially HIV.

You do not wish to inform any of your sexual partners of this diagnosis as you're embarrassed, however if encouraged and offered the anonymous service you accept.

## Examiner Instructions

The candidate is a Foundation Year Doctor in the Genitourinary Medicine (GUM) clinic. Frank is a 19-year-old man who has presented after receiving a text telling him that he's been in contact with someone who has Chlamydia. The candidate has been asked to take a focused history and counsel him about how this will be managed,

They do not need to examine the patient.

**Mark Scheme**

| Task | Achieved | Not Achieved |
|---|---|---|
| Introduces self, washes hands | | |
| Confirms name, age & occupation of patient | | |
| Establishes reason for consultation | | |
| Sensitively explains the patient may have contracted chlamydia, discusses text service | | |
| Clarifies what the patient currently knows about chlamydia, explains what this is | | |
| Gives warning shot re. sensitive questions and reiterates confidentiality | | |
| Asks about sexual partners in last 6 months: gender, type of sex and contraceptive use | | |
| Asks about high risk behaviour for HIV/Hepatitis e.g. IVDU, travel, background of partner | | |
| Asks if they have paid for or been paid for sex | | |
| Asks about presence of any symptoms but reiterates may be asymptomatic | | |
| Offer screening of other STIs, including HIV | | |
| Offer empirical treatment (1g Azithromycin stat) | | |
| Discusses how to avoid reinfection – avoid sexual contact until 1 week post treatment | | |
| Encourages partner notification from last 3 months | | |
| Discuss options of disclosure e.g. anonymous text service, personally informing | | |
| Encourages regular STI checks with change of sexual partner | | |
| | | |
| Identifies patient's ideas, concerns and expectations in an empathetic manner | | |
| Summarises key points, checks understanding & avoids jargon | | |
| Suggests follow up or take home information about contraception | | |
| Completes station in a confident and professional manner | | |
| | | |
| Examiners Global Mark | /5 | |
| Actors Global Mark | /5 | |
| Total Station Mark | /30 | |

# Learning points

- It is important to remain non-judgemental and supportive of those who come forward following contract tracing. It is an increasingly common infection, with reports of 70% of people with chlamydia under 25 (*Nwokolo et al, 2015*), many of whom are asymptomatic and undiagnosed.

- Chlamydia may remain asymptomatic can be found by chance at routine STI screening however in women symptoms of lower abdominal pain, dysuria, vaginal discharge and intermenstrual or post coital bleeding may occur.

- Encourage the patient that contact tracing is anonymous and prevents ongoing spread, which can be exponential. The 'look-back' period should be 6 months for those that have been asymptomatic.

## Station 33: Discussing Pelvic Inflammatory Disease

## Candidate Instructions

You are the Foundation Year Doctor in a GP surgery. Claire is a 26-year-old woman who was diagnosed with pelvic inflammatory disease a few days ago when she attended the Emergency Department feeling unwell. She has been given medication and is now feeling better, but has come to discuss the implications of this diagnosis. Please take a brief history and counsel her about the potential long-term impact of this diagnosis.

You do not need to examine the patient.

You have eight minutes.

## Actor Instructions

You are Claire, a 26-year-old bank clerk. You have come to speak with the GP today about the implications of your recent diagnosis of pelvic inflammatory disease (PID). Last week you were feeling generally unwell with lower abdominal and back pain and a funny discharge. You were seen in the Emergency Department and examined by the gynaecology team, who diagnosed PID and gave you two antibiotics that you have now completed. You were concerned that something was wrong for the past few weeks as you noticed it was quite uncomfortable when you had sex, which does not usually happen.

You have a past history of chlamydia and gonorrhoea. You cannot remember if you finished the course of antibiotics, and you admit you are awful at taking tablets. You have had unprotected sexual intercourse in the last six months with three different sexual partners. You have no other medical problems.

You are worried about the diagnosis and have come to see your GP. You have been reading about the effects of PID on your long-term health and your future fertility, and thus, wanted to get some information from your own doctor about this.

# Examiner Instructions

The candidate is a Foundation Year Doctor in a GP practice. Claire is a 26-year-old woman who was diagnosed with pelvic inflammatory disease a few days ago when she attended the Emergency Department feeling unwell. She has been given medication and is now feeling better, but has come to discuss the implications of this diagnosis. The candidate has been asked to take a brief history and counsel her about the potential long-term impact of this diagnosis.

They do not need to examine the patient.

**Mark Scheme**

| Task | Achieved | Not Achieved |
|---|---|---|
| Introduces self, washes hands | | |
| Confirms name, age & occupation of patient | | |
| Establishes reason for consultation | | |
| | | |
| Takes brief history of recent symptoms leading to A&E attendance | | |
| Asks brief sexual and gynaecological history | | |
| Discusses treatment regime and compliance | | |
| Asks patient what they understand about PID | | |
| Explains development of PID – tracking from vagina to upper reproductive tract | | |
| Explains infection can lead to a collection of pus in the pelvis causing dyspareunia and pain | | |
| Explains the causes are usually STIs | | |
| Explains long-term complications of PID | | |
| Explain symptoms of chronic PID | | |
| Explains risk of abscesses and perihepatitis | | |
| Explains increased risk of infertility and ectopic pregnancy with each acute episode of PID | | |
| Explains process of contact tracing and treatment for partner | | |
| Reiterates importance of barrier protection with new partners | | |
| | | |
| Identifies patient's ideas, concerns and expectations in an empathetic manner | | |
| Summarises key points, checks understanding & avoids jargon | | |
| Suggests follow up or take home information | | |
| Completes station in a confident and professional manner | | |
| | | |
| Examiners Global Mark | /5 | |
| Actors Global Mark | /5 | |
| Total Station Mark | /30 | |

## Learning points

- Pelvic inflammatory disease (PID) is an umbrella term for infection of the upper female genital tract, including the uterus, Fallopian tubes, and ovaries. PID usually results from ascending infection from the cervix.

- The commonest causes of PID are chlamydia and gonorrhoea. Though less common, there are also non-sexually transmitted diseases such as Gardnerella vaginalis, If an episode of PID follows uterine instrumentation (e.g. surgical TOP, ERPC, IUD insertion), it is usually due to non-sexually transmitted bacteria.

- As with most illness there is a severity spectrum for PID. Mild or moderate disease can be managed in primary care or outpatients, whereas more severe and systemic disease will require hospital admission for intravenous antibiotics.

# Station 34: Unwanted Pregnancy

## Candidate Instructions

You are the Foundation Year Doctor in a GP surgery. Avanti is a 24-year-old woman who has requested an urgent appointment as she has recently discovered she is pregnant. Please discuss the patient's concerns and how she wishes to proceed with the pregnancy.

You do not need to examine the patient.

You have eight minutes.

## Actor Instructions

You are Avanti, a 24-year-old singer/songwriter. You have come to speak with the GP today after noticing your period was two weeks late. You did a home pregnancy test yesterday and have discovered that you are pregnant. You are in a new relationship and use condoms with your boyfriend, but admit that there have been a few accidents. You are quite upset as you have a number of concerns. You do not think either of you are ready for a baby, and your career is just starting to take off and you cannot afford to put this on hold right now. You and your partner are not financially secure, and you would not have the support of your conservative and deeply religious family.

Whilst you do wish to have children one day, you do not feel it is the right time and you cannot continue with the pregnancy. You have not told your partner, but your best friend is very supportive and you can confide in her.

You wish to know what your options are for termination, and would like this done as soon as possible. You are worried that leaving it too late will mean it cannot be done or you will start to show.

You have not had an STI check but will accept one if offered.

Your last menstrual period was 6 weeks ago. You have had no discharge, bleeding or pain. You have never had an STI as far as you are aware. You are otherwise fit and well, and do not smoke. You drink 2-3 glasses of wine a week, but not since finding out about the pregnancy.

## Examiner Instructions

The candidate is a Foundation Year Doctor in a GP practice. Avanti is a 24-year-old woman who has requested an urgent appointment as she has recently discovered she is pregnant. The candidate has been asked to discuss the patient's concerns and how she wishes to proceed with the pregnancy.

They do not need to examine the patient.

**Mark Scheme**

| Task | Achieved | Not Achieved |
|---|---|---|
| Introduces self, washes hands | | |
| Confirms name, age & occupation of patient | | |
| Establishes reason for consultation | | |
| | | |
| Asks open questions about patient's feelings towards the pregnancy | | |
| Asks about factors impacting decision: personal, financial, social, family & professional | | |
| Asks if partner is aware or if they have a support network | | |
| Discusses alternative option to TOP: adoption | | |
| Asks about LMP and estimates gestation | | |
| Asks brief gynaecological and medical history | | |
| Discusses/offers STI check | | |
| Explains medical procedure & indications | | |
| Explains surgical procedure & indications | | |
| Discusses complications of pregnancy – Bleeding, infection, physical/mental trauma | | |
| Explains that blood test required to check rhesus status as she may need Anti-D injection | | |
| Discusses process of referring for termination | | |
| Offers time to think about options or counselling services via family planning clinics | | |
| | | |
| Identifies patient's ideas, concerns and expectations in an empathetic manner | | |
| Summarises key points, checks understanding & avoids jargon | | |
| Suggests follow up or take home information | | |
| Completes station in a confident and professional manner | | |
| | | |
| Examiners Global Mark | /5 | |
| Actors Global Mark | /5 | |
| Total Station Mark | /30 | |

## Learning points

- This is a difficult conversation and decision to make for the majority of patients. Encourage them to seek support from partner / friends / family and/or offer counselling to help make the decision.

- The Human Fertilisation & Embryology Act 1990 (*HFEA, 1990*) states the current law allows termination of pregnancy to be granted if:

a.	Pregnancy is <24 weeks and risk of injury to physical/mental health of woman or existing children in the family greater if it is continued than if it is terminated.
b.	Termination is necessary to prevent grave permanent injury to physical/mental health of pregnant woman.
c.	Pregnancy at any stage would involve risk to the life of the pregnant woman greater if it is continued than if it is terminated.
d.	Substantial risk of severe mental/physical abnormalities in the unborn child causing serious handicap.

- Remember to offer an STI check and follow-up to discuss contraceptive options. Often at the time of a surgical TOP, an IUD can be placed. Following a medical TOP, several methods including the OCP, depot or implant can be started on the day of prostaglandin administration. The IUD can be inserted following the next menstrual cycle.

# Station 35: Early Miscarriage

## Candidate Instructions

You are the Foundation Year Doctor in the Early Pregnancy Assessment Unit. Cassie is a 22-year-old woman who is 10 weeks pregnant and experienced some moderate bleeding with clots and abdominal cramping today, which has now settled. An ultrasound performed revealed that there was no fetal heartbeat and a closed cervical os but with remaining tissue in the uterus. Please explain these findings to her and answer any questions she may have.

You do not need to examine the patient.

You have eight minutes

## Actor Instructions

You are Cassie, a 22-year-old social media blogger. You have come to the Early Pregnancy Assessment Unit after some moderate bleeding with clots and abdominal cramping today, which has now settled. You are 10 weeks pregnant and you are very scared that the baby is in danger. This is your first pregnancy with your childhood sweetheart and you are both very excited. Your partner is unfortunately out of town and you are at the clinic alone.

You have just had an ultrasound and are here to get the results. If the candidate asks if you have anyone with you, say no but you are keen to find out now as you are worried it is bad news. This shows that you have had a miscarriage, which the candidate will inform you of. You are understandably upset by this and want to know the answers to the following questions:

- Why has this happened?
- Is this my fault?
- What will happen now? Do I need treatment for this?
- (If not addressed) - I was told that I am Rhesus negative at my booking visit and I would need injections if I had bleeding in pregnancy, do I need to have one now?

## Examiner Instructions

The candidate is the Foundation Year Doctor in the Early Pregnancy Assessment Unit. Cassie is a 22-year-old woman who is 10 weeks pregnant and experienced some moderate bleeding with clots and abdominal cramping today, which has now settled. An ultrasound performed revealed that there was no fetal heartbeat and a closed cervical os but with remaining tissue in the uterus. They have been asked to explain these findings to her and answer any questions she may have.

They do not need to examine the patient.

**Mark Scheme**

| Task | Achieved | Not Achieved |
|---|---|---|
| Introduces self, washes hands | | |
| Confirms name, age & occupation of patient | | |
| Establishes reason for consultation | | |
| | | |
| Asks if patient has somebody with her to discuss the results of the scan, gives warning shot | | |
| Takes a brief history including parity & gestation | | |
| Sensitively explains results of ultrasound scan | | |
| Gives time to the patient to absorb and appropriate silences | | |
| Explains that miscarriages are common in early pregnancy | | |
| Gives examples of causes for early miscarriage | | |
| Reassures that it is not preventable and not caused by anything she has done | | |
| Discusses management options for incomplete miscarriage | | |
| Explains the options of expectant management with benefits and risks | | |
| Explains the option of medical management with benefits and risks | | |
| Explains the option of surgical management with benefits and risks | | |
| Discusses prognosis for future pregnancies | | |
| Discusses anti-D advice – not required unless surgical management undertaken as she is 10 weeks pregnancy | | |
| | | |
| Identifies patient's ideas, concerns and expectations in an empathetic manner | | |
| Summarises key points, checks understanding & avoids jargon | | |
| Suggests follow up or take home information | | |
| Completes station in a confident and professional manner | | |
| | | |
| Examiners Global Mark | /5 | |
| Actors Global Mark | /5 | |
| Total Station Mark | /30 | |

## Learning points

- This is a difficult time for the patient and their partner, and in the early weeks prior to a booking scan they may not have shared the news of the pregnancy with anyone else. In most cases they are young and fit and have no medical problems and so the loss of the pregnancy can seem hard to believe. It is important to reiterate that we do not have measures to prevent the miscarriage once it has begun and that it is not due to 'any fault' of theirs.

- If the patient has experienced 3 or more spontaneous miscarriages in succession, this is classed as 'recurrent' miscarriage and should be referred for investigation. This can be a result of anatomical abnormalities, infection, chromosomal defects or antiphosphalipid syndrome (*Impey, 2012*)

- Anti D is administered at any sensitising event (*Qureshi et al., 2014*) This includes:

  - Before 12 weeks: ectopic or molar pregnancy, significant, repeated or painful bleeding, surgical TOP
  - After 12 weeks: invasive antenatal procedures, antepartum haemorrhage, abdominal trauma, external cephalic version, intrauterine death, stillbirth or live birth

# Station 36: Antenatal Scanning

## Candidate Instructions

You are the Foundation Year Doctor in a GP surgery. Thea is a 25-year-old woman who is 7 weeks pregnant with her first baby. She has asked to speak to you following her booking visit with the midwife about her upcoming antenatal scans and investigations. Please counsel the woman about routine antenatal scans and discuss her concerns.

You do not need to take a full history or examine the patient.

You have eight minutes.

## Actor Instructions

You are Thea, a 25-year-old office worker. You have asked to speak with the GP about the antenatal scans available in pregnancy. You have just seen the midwife for your booking visit and she explained a bit about the blood tests, routine ultrasounds at 12 and 20 weeks and general health advice about diet and supplements.

This is your first pregnancy and you are 7 weeks in. You are very excited about being pregnant and have had a great experience so far with only mild morning sickness. You are planning on having the baby on your own as the father does not want to be involved, but you have supportive mum who is willing to help raise the baby with you.

You are anxious to know about Down's syndrome testing as your younger brother has this condition. You love your brother very much but you have seen how much your mum has gone through. If you were told your baby had Down's syndrome you would consider an abortion (feel free to get very emotional when explaining this).

If the candidate asks you can give a very basic history but try to steer the patient away from taking a detailed history. You have never been pregnant before. You do not drink alcohol or smoke. You are fit and well with no medical problems or allergies and you take folic acid. The midwife told you that you were low risk at your booking visit and would be receiving midwife led care.

You have some specific questions:
- What routine scans will I get in my pregnancy?
- What conditions can be screened for in pregnancy?
- How can I be sure my baby will not have Down's syndrome?
- What tests are available to diagnose this?
- Are there any risks to the tests?
- What happens if it is confirmed?
- What can make me more likely to have a child with Down's syndrome

## Examiner Instructions

A 25-year-old woman who is 7 weeks pregnant has come to the surgery following her booking visit with the midwife. The candidate is a Foundation Year Doctor who has been asked to counsel the woman about the upcoming routine antenatal investigations.

The candidate does not need to take a full obstetric history as in the booking visit.

**Mark Scheme**

| Task | Achieved | Not Achieved |
|---|---|---|
| Introduces self, washes hands | | |
| Confirms name, age & occupation of patient | | |
| Establishes reason for consultation | | |
| | | |
| Establishes patient's current knowledge of antenatal testing | | |
| Explains routine ultrasound scans: 12 & 20 weeks | | |
| 12 week scan is 'dating' scan – can detect spina bifida | | |
| 20 week scan is 'anomaly' scan | | |
| Explains role of blood tests – can detect blood disorders if high risk, can indicate Down's risk | | |
| Discusses risk factors for Down's syndrome | | |
| Discusses diagnostic testing – amniocentesis or CVS and differences between these | | |
| Discusses associated risks of diagnostic tests | | |
| Discusses options if Down's syndrome or other disorder is confirmed | | |
| Maintains non-judgemental attitude when discussing option of termination if desired | | |
| Elicits source of patients concerns (family history and personal experience) | | |
| Asks about support network | | |
| Reassures that there is no increased risk because of family history | | |
| | | |
| Identifies patient's ideas, concerns and expectations in an empathetic manner | | |
| Summarises key points, checks understanding & avoids jargon | | |
| Suggests follow up or take home information | | |
| Completes station in a confident and professional manner | | |
| | | |
| Examiners Global Mark | /5 | |
| Actors Global Mark | /5 | |
| Total Station Mark | /30 | |

## Learning points

- The risk of Down's syndrome increases with maternal age – divide by 3 for every 5 years after 35. 1/300 at 35, 1/100 at 40, 1/50 at 45.

- The initial 12-week scan is to confirm dates, location of pregnancy and check nuchal translucency. The 20-week scan is known as the anomaly scan that assesses for physical abnormalities.

- Remember to always be non-judgemental with women seeking possible terminations, regardless of your personal views. Always provide people with all options available, and facilitate this if you are not directly able to provide this service yourself.

# Station 37: Sickle Cell in Pregnancy

## Candidate Instructions

You are the Foundation Year Doctor at a GP surgery. You have been asked to see Gloria, a 25-year-old Nigerian woman who is intending on starting a family. She is a known carrier of sickle cell disease and would like to discuss how this will impact her pregnancy. Please counsel her and discuss her concerns.

You do not need to examine the patient.

You have eight minutes.

## Actor Instructions

You are Gloria, a 25-year-old typist. You have presented to the GP today to discuss your concerns about starting a family with your husband. You are both from Nigeria and you are aware that you are a sickle cell carrier, although your husband has never been tested. You are worried about having children because of the risk of passing on the disease, and are also worried about the effect this may have on your pregnancy.

Your mother has sickle cell disease and has suffered with severe pain and has had frequent admissions for pain relief. Both you and your sister are carriers. You have never had any complications as a result of being a carrier and you are otherwise well. You do not really know much about how sickle cell is inherited, or what causes the disease.

You have some specific concerns about sickle cell disease:
1.  What is sickle cell disease? What is the difference between having the disease and being a carrier?
2.  Will my child have sickle cell disease?
3.  Does it affect my chances of becoming pregnant?
4.  How can you test my baby for sickle cell disease?
5.  What happens if my baby has sickle cell disease?

## Examiner Instructions

The candidate is a Foundation Year Doctor in a GP surgery. They have been asked to see Gloria, a 25-year-old Nigerian woman who is intending on starting a family. She is a known carrier of sickle cell disease about would like to discuss how this will impact her pregnancy and risks. They have been asked to counsel her and discuss her concerns.

They do not need to examine the patient.

**Mark Scheme**

| Task | Achieved | Not Achieved |
|---|---|---|
| Introduces self, washes hands | | |
| Confirms name, age & occupation of patient | | |
| Establishes reason for consultation | | |
| | | |
| Checks current knowledge of sickle cell disease | | |
| Explains the difference between sickle cell disease and trait | | |
| Establishes patient is a sickle cell carrier – asks about family history and symptoms | | |
| Asks about her husband's sickle cell status | | |
| Explains that it is an autosomal recessive condition and the pattern of inheritance | | |
| Discusses disease/trait inheritance probability if partner is a carrier or not | | |
| Suggests partner screening if status unknown | | |
| Suggests importance of antenatal screening for other haemoglobinopathies | | |
| Explains implications if the child develops sickle cell disease | | |
| Explains implications if the child is a sickle cell carrier | | |
| Explains diagnostic techniques in pregnancy if the mother wishes to confirm this | | |
| Explains newborn bloodspot testing | | |
| Explains importance of antenatal booking visit | | |
| | | |
| Identifies patient's ideas, concerns and expectations in an empathetic manner | | |
| Summarises key points, checks understanding & avoids jargon | | |
| Suggests follow up or take home information | | |
| Completes station in a confident and professional manner | | |
| | | |
| Examiners Global Mark | /5 | |
| Actors Global Mark | /5 | |
| Total Station Mark | /30 | |

## Learning points

- It is useful to have a framework for explaining the inheritance patterns for autosomal recessive and dominant conditions. Remember you can use diagrams to help explain.

- All newborn babies are offered a heel prick blood spot test 5-7 days after birth, but mothers may choose to undergo antenatal genetic screening and amniocentesis and chorionic villus sampling (CVS) are diagnostic in pregnancy.

- Routine partner screening is offered to mothers who are known to be sickle cell carriers. If both parents are carriers they will be offered the chance to definitively test the fetus by chorionic villus sampling or Amniocentesis between 0-15 weeks gestation.

## Station 38: Whooping Cough Vaccination in Pregnancy

## Candidate Instructions

You are the Foundation Year Doctor at a GP surgery. Heidi is a 30-year-old pregnant woman who has made an appointment to discuss the whooping cough vaccination. Please counsel her about the vaccination and discuss any concerns she may have.

You do not need to examine the patient.

You have eight minutes.

## Actor Instructions

You are Heidi, a 30-year-old lawyer. You are 19 weeks pregnant with your first child. You have come to see the GP today because you were told to book an appointment to have your whooping cough vaccine next week. You were fully up to date with your own childhood vaccinations and do not understand why you need to have another one now, especially while you are pregnant.

This is your second pregnancy, but your first ended in miscarriage at 6 weeks. Whilst no cause for the miscarriage was found, you are still concerned about this pregnancy and the risk of having another miscarriage, despite being reassured that it is unlikely. You have no other health problems and took folic acid until you were 12 weeks.

You do not know what whooping cough is, and want to know if the vaccine is a) necessary and b) safe in pregnancy. You are concerned that every few years new data emerges about different vaccines and are worried this may turn out to be dangerous. You have been careful not to take any other medication and having been eating well to optimise your health. You want to keep this pregnancy as natural as possible and don't want to feel pushed into having the vaccine without understanding the risks. You are also concerned that you may get the disease from the vaccination.

You have some questions you would like answered (if not already addressed):

- Can I get the disease from the vaccine?
- Can the vaccine harm the baby?
- Does this mean the baby will not need their immunisations at 8 weeks for whooping cough?
- If I decide not to have the vaccine, will this affect my follow up and interactions with the midwife?

At the end of the consultation, you are still not sure about your decision but would like to think about it and come back

## Examiner Instructions

The candidate is a Foundation Year Doctor in a GP surgery. They have been asked to see Heidi, a 30-year-old woman who is 19 weeks pregnant and would like to discuss the whooping cough vaccination. They have been asked to counsel her about the vaccination and the indications and discuss her concerns.

They do not need to examine the patient.

**Mark Scheme**

| Task | Achieved | Not Achieved |
|---|---|---|
| Introduces self, washes hands | | |
| Confirms name, age & occupation of patient | | |
| Establishes reason for consultation | | |
| | | |
| Checks current knowledge of whooping cough and the vaccination, elicits concerns | | |
| Explains what whooping cough/pertussis is and complications | | |
| Discusses risk in young babies before immunisation, more likely to need admission | | |
| Informs patient it is recommended nationally | | |
| Discusses side effects of vaccine, no known contraindications | | |
| Explains not a 'live' vaccine – therefore cannot get the disease from vaccination | | |
| Explains when the vaccine is recommended in pregnancy (from 20 weeks up to 32 weeks) | | |
| Explains it is less effective later in pregnancy, but can be give up until labour | | |
| Advises that the baby still needs vaccination as part of their immunisation schedule after birth | | |
| Advises she can make an informed decision | | |
| Reassures patient that she will continue to be supported by staff regardless of her choice | | |
| Advises patient to discuss this with her partner/support network/antenatal group | | |
| | | |
| Gives clear recommended advice in a non-judgemental and non-coercive manner | | |
| Identifies patient's ideas, concerns and expectations in an empathetic manner | | |
| Summarises key points, checks understanding & avoids jargon | | |
| Suggests follow up or take home information | | |
| Completes station in a confident and professional manner | | |
| Examiners Global Mark | /5 | |
| Actors Global Mark | /5 | |
| Total Station Mark | /30 | |

# Learning points

- There is no known evidence to date that the vaccine is unsafe in pregnancy. It is important to confidently reiterate this to patients so that they can be assured that this is a national clinical recommendation and research to support this. Specifically, there was no increased risk in stillbirth seen in an observational study of over 20 000 women given the vaccine in pregnancy (*Donegan et al, 2014*).

- In the UK there is no whooping cough-only vaccine, the vaccine you'll be given also protects against polio, diphtheria and tetanus. The vaccine is similar to the 4-in-1 vaccine – the pre-school booster that's routinely given to children before they start school.

- Any discussions regarding pregnancy or childhood vaccinations can be difficult if parents have strong views against vaccines. As a health professional, it is important to given unbiased, factual information in order to allow patients to make an informed decision. Excellent patient information leaflets exist that should be given to parents so they can digest the facts in their own time in a less pressured environment. Follow up appointments should be made with their GPs to discuss it further

-

# Station 39: Chickenpox in Pregnancy

## Candidate Instructions

You are the Foundation Year Doctor at a GP surgery. You have been asked to see Arpita, a 32-year-old woman who is 15 weeks pregnant with her second child. She has come to see you as her nephew has just developed chicken pox. Please counsel her about the implications of contact with chicken pox in pregnancy and discuss her concerns.

You do not need to examine the patient.

You have eight minutes.

## Actor Instructions

You are Arpita, a 32-year-old radio programme director. You are 15 weeks pregnant with your second child. You have come to see the GP today because your nephew who you saw 3 days ago has been diagnosed with chickenpox. You are concerned because you cannot remember if you have had chickenpox or the vaccination and you have been told it might affect the baby.

You spent the day taking your nephew to the zoo and had lots of close physical contact with him that day. He was a bit grumpy and had lost his appetite so you had tried to make him feel better with lots of cuddles. He came out in the rash yesterday and your sister took him to the doctor who said it was chicken pox.

Your pregnancy is progressing well. You had your first scan a couple of weeks ago and there were no issues. Your morning sickness has mostly resolved. You have no other health issues. Your daughter who is 3 was also with you at the zoo. She has never had chicken pox either but has not been unwell as yet.

You would like to know what the risks are for your baby and if you need any test or tablets. If VZIG injection is recommended, you are not keen to have straightaway as you have a needle phobia.

Please ask the following questions if not answered by the candidate:
- Do I have to have the injection now or can I think about it and come back?
- What are the risks to the baby? Could I lose the baby?
- How can I prevent this happening again if get pregnant in the future?

# Examiner Instructions

The candidate is a Foundation Year Doctor in a GP surgery. They have been asked to see Arpita, a 32-year-old woman who is 15 weeks pregnant with her second child. She has come to see the doctor as her nephew has just developed chicken pox. They have been asked to counsel her about the implications of contact with chicken pox in pregnancy and discuss her concerns.

They do not need to examine the patient.

## Mark Scheme

| Task | Achieved | Not Achieved |
|---|---|---|
| Introduces self, washes hands | | |
| Confirms name, age & occupation of patient | | |
| Establishes reason for consultation | | |
| | | |
| Checks current knowledge of chickenpox | | |
| Determines level of contact with affected child | | |
| Clarifies immunity status | | |
| Explains risks to fetal health | | |
| Explains risks to mother's health | | |
| Discusses varicella zoster immune globulin (VZIG) injection | | |
| Advises can be given ≤10 days after contact if no symptoms – ineffective once blisters appear | | |
| Advises if develops chickenpox, patient would be referred to fetal medicine | | |
| Advises treatment with aciclovir if develops chickenpox | | |
| Safety netting – seek help if severe symptoms, breathing problems or immunosuppressed | | |
| Advises that risk of miscarriage is not increased prior to 28 weeks | | |
| Discusses option of postpartum vaccination | | |
| Advises against getting pregnant 3 months after vaccination | | |
| | | |
| Identifies patient's ideas, concerns and expectations in an empathetic manner | | |
| Summarises key points, checks understanding & avoids jargon | | |
| Suggests follow up or take home information | | |
| Completes station in a confident and professional manner | | |
| | | |
| Examiners Global Mark | /5 | |
| Actors Global Mark | /5 | |
| Total Station Mark | /30 | |

## Learning points

- Important to check the immunity of the woman as 90% women who have had chickenpox previously will be immune and do not need the VZIG injection

- It is important to allow the mother to come to her own decision with a full understanding of the risks. The VZIG injection can be given up to 10 days after exposure providing that no blisters have appeared, so it is possible to compromise and offer follow up to revisit the discussion in the next few days.

- Pregnant mothers who have had recent steroids, chronic lung disease, pregnancy over 20 weeks or smoke cigarettes are at increased risk of developing the disease (*RCOG, 2008*).

# Station 40: Hypertension and Proteinuria in Pregnancy

## Candidate Instructions

You are the Foundation Year Doctor in the Maternity Assessment Unit. You have been asked to see Agnes, a 35-year-old woman who is 33 weeks pregnant with twins and has been referred by her GP as her blood pressure has been found to be higher than usual. The nurse in the unit has recorded this in the triage notes:

Blood Pressure is 170/100
Urine dipstick: +++ protein.

Please counsel her about the implications of this and discuss her concerns.

You do not need to examine the patient.

You have eight minutes.

# Actor Instructions

You are Agnes, a 35-year-old medical secretary. You are 33 weeks pregnant with twins and have been referred to the Maternity Triage Unit by your GP as he was concerned about your blood pressure. You are informed about the results of your urine dip and blood pressure reading today, and this indicates an abnormal finding.

Over the past week, you have noticed some swelling around the feet and ankles. Initially, you felt it was just a normal side effect of pregnancy but over the last two days you have noticed some swelling of your hands and wrists as well and your watch and wedding ring feel uncomfortable. In addition to this, you have noticed headaches over the past two days, which are not eased by Paracetamol. You have had no blurring of your vision, and you do not feel more breathless than usual and have had no chest or tummy pain. You have not noticed any frothing of your urine. You visited the GP because of these symptoms and he referred you to the Maternity Unit because your blood pressure was higher than usual and warranted a specialist opinion.

This is your first pregnancy and has been otherwise uncomplicated and you have felt well and remained active throughout. You have not had any issues with your blood pressure so far, but you did miss your last midwife appointment at 31 weeks as you were on holiday. You have had no previous miscarriages or abortions. You have no past medical history, and you are not on regular medications and have no allergies. You live with your husband and do not drink alcohol or smoke.

If asked about family history, your mother died in her 50s from breast cancer. She had 2 early caesarean deliveries for 'complications' but you are not sure why.

You are very anxious as to what the high blood pressure means for the babies and you are also concerned about your symptoms of swelling and headache as you have never had these before.

## Examiner Instructions

The candidate is a Foundation Year Doctor in the Maternity Assessment Unit. They have been asked to see Agnes, a 35-year-old woman who is 33 weeks pregnant with twins and has been referred by her GP as her blood pressure has been found to be higher than usual. The nurse in the unit has recorded this in the triage notes:

Blood Pressure is 170/100
Urine dipstick: +++ protein.

They have been asked to counsel her about the implications of this and discuss her concerns.

They do not need to examine the patient.

**Mark Scheme**

| Task | Achieved | Not Achieved |
|---|---|---|
| Introduces self, washes hands | | |
| Confirms name, age & occupation of patient | | |
| Establishes reason for consultation | | |
| | | |
| Asks about headaches, confusion or visual changes/blurring | | |
| Asks about shortness of breath and/or oedema | | |
| Asks about urine output, colour and/or frothing | | |
| Asks about abdominal pain | | |
| Elicits past medical history, drug history including allergies | | |
| Elicits previous obstetric history and history of current pregnancy | | |
| Identifies risk factors for pre-eclampsia (first pregnancy, twins, possible family history) | | |
| Sensitively explains likely diagnosis of pre-eclampsia and explains what this is | | |
| Discusses investigations (bloods, urinalysis, USS) | | |
| Discusses aims of management – reduce BP | | |
| Explains will require admission until blood pressure controlled | | |
| Explains may need to deliver early if not controlled or symptoms worsening | | |
| Discusses complications if BP not controlled | | |
| | | |
| Identifies patient's ideas, concerns and expectations in an empathetic manner | | |
| Summarises key points, checks understanding & avoids jargon | | |
| Suggests follow up or take home information | | |
| Completes station in a confident and professional manner | | |
| | | |
| Examiners Global Mark | /5 | |
| Actors Global Mark | /5 | |
| Total Station Mark | /30 | |

## Learning points

- Fetal complications of pre-eclampsia include IUGR, prematurity, placental abruption and hypoxia and increased risk of mortality (*Impey,, 2012*)

- Maternal complications of pre-eclampsia include eclampsia, HELLP syndrome, DIC, end organ failure and cerebral haemorrhage if left untreated.

- Hypertension in pregnancy requires postnatal follow up. If persistently abnormal at 6 weeks, this may warrant referral to secondary care.

# Station 41: Gestational Diabetes

## Candidate Instructions

You are the Foundation Year Doctor in the Antenatal Clinic. You have been asked to speak to Anna, a 32-year-old pregnant woman, about the results of her oral glucose tolerance test.

Results:

Fasting value:     6.9mmol/L
2 hours post-test:12.3mmol/L


Please explain these results to the patient, and discuss management and complications associated with this diagnosis.

You do not need to examine the patient

You have eight minutes.

## Actor Instructions

You are Anna, a 32-year-old newsreader. You have come to the Antenatal Clinic today for the results of your oral glucose tolerance test. You are 13 weeks pregnant with your first baby and so far have been feeling well and morning sickness has settled down. You had a blood test at your GP surgery which showed your sugar level was a little on the higher side and they sent you for an OGTT.

This is your first pregnancy, which took a while to conceive as you have polycystic ovaries with irregular periods. You have no other medical problems, and you are not on any medication and you have no allergies.

You are overweight, but have struggled to control your eating habits and have admittedly been 'eating for two'. You do not drink or smoke.

Questions:
- What does this mean for you and your baby?
- You are worried as you have heard that Diabetes can cause all sorts of risks to the baby but now that the damage is done, is there anything you can do to stop this?
- You are not keen to take medications as you are worried about the risk to the baby, is there any way to do this drug free and just control your diet?
- Will this mean you will continue to have diabetes after the baby is born?

## Examiner Instructions

The candidate is a Foundation Year Doctor in the Antenatal Clinic. They have been asked to speak to Anna, a 32-year-old pregnant woman, about the results of her oral glucose tolerance test.

Results:

Fasting value:      6.9mmol/L
2 hours post-test:12.3mmol/L

The candidate has been asked to explain these results to the patient and discuss management and complications associated with this diagnosis.

They do not need to examine the patient.

**Mark Scheme**

| Task | Achieved | Not Achieved |
|---|---|---|
| Introduces self, washes hands | | |
| Confirms name, age & occupation of patient | | |
| Establishes reason for consultation | | |
| | | |
| Identifies what the patient knows so far about the OGTT | | |
| Explains results of OGTT | | |
| Correctly identifies a diagnosis of GDM | | |
| Checks patient's understanding of what GDM is | | |
| Outlines risks in pregnancy and delivery | | |
| Outlines risks to foetus before and after birth | | |
| Outlines maternal health risks if uncontrolled | | |
| Stresses importance of tight glucose control in pregnancy to reduce risks | | |
| Recommends diet control and low sugar intake | | |
| Discusses treatment – drug treatment strongly recommended due to benefit vs risk | | |
| Explain the patient will be monitored by the hospital obstetrics team due to increased risk | | |
| Informs patient testing will be repeated 6 weeks post-partum to check if sugars normalised | | |
| Explains increased risk of GDM in future pregnancy and DM in later life | | |
| | | |
| Identifies patient's ideas, concerns and expectations in an empathetic manner | | |
| Summarises key points, checks understanding & avoids jargon | | |
| Suggests follow up or take home information | | |
| Completes station in a confident and professional manner | | |
| | | |
| Examiners Global Mark | /5 | |
| Actors Global Mark | /5 | |
| Total Station Mark | /30 | |

## Learning points

- NICE recommend that diagnosis of GDM should be made if:

  Fasting plasma glucose level of 5.6 mmol/L or above, or 2-hour plasma glucose level of 7.8 mmol/L or above.

- Foetal complications of diabetes include macrosomia, prematurity, congenital abnormalities and birth trauma or complications for both mother and baby.

- GDM is becoming more and more prevalent and is associated with serious risks. It is important to counsel women who are high risk before getting pregnant to lose weight and reduce sugar intake to prevent GDM wherever possible.

# Station 42: Antenatal Diagnosis of Down's Syndrome

## Candidate Instructions

You are the Foundation Year Doctor in the Antenatal Clinic. You have been asked to speak to Sofia, a 37-year-old pregnant woman who has been informed that her unborn baby has Down's syndrome following diagnostic testing. Please discuss her concerns and answer any questions she may have.

You do not need to examine the patient

You have eight minutes

## Actor Instructions

You are Sofia, a 37-year-old store manager and you are 17 weeks pregnant with your second child. You have come to the Antenatal Clinic for follow up after receiving the news that your unborn child has Down's syndrome. You had amniocentesis screening one week ago that confirmed this. This has come as a shock to you, and you and your husband are devastated.

Since the test, you have had slight twinges but no bleeding, fevers or discharge. You are otherwise feeling well, and you think you may be feeling 'flutters' from the baby moving.

You are in two minds as to whether you wish to continue with the pregnancy or not, but you wanted to find out about the complications of Down's syndrome and coping as a family. You have a friend who has a son with Down's syndrome and they are always in and out of hospital because he has a heart problem, and you are scared this will be too much for your family to cope with.

Questions you would like answered include:

- How certain are the test results, is there a chance they could be wrong?
- What is Down's syndrome? How does it affect the baby?
- Are they going to die early?
- What if we choose to terminate the pregnancy? Is that still possible at 17 weeks?
- What is the likelihood of having another child with Down's syndrome?

## Examiner Instructions

The candidate is a Foundation Year Doctor in the Antenatal Clinic. They have been asked to speak to Sofia, a 37-year-old pregnant woman, who has been informed that her unborn baby has Down's syndrome following diagnostic testing. The candidate has been asked to discuss her concerns and answer any questions she may have.

They do not need to examine the patient.

**Mark Scheme**

| Task | Achieved | Not Achieved |
|---|---|---|
| Introduces self, washes hands | | |
| Confirms name, age & occupation of patient | | |
| Establishes reason for consultation | | |
| | | |
| Asks about how patient feels since last meeting | | |
| Appropriate use of silence and active listening | | |
| Discuss support network and if patient has had anyone to talk to about diagnosis | | |
| Specify the results of amniocentesis are definitive in 98-99% cases | | |
| Establishes patient's current knowledge of Down's Syndrome | | |
| Specifies risk of Down's syndrome pregnancy increases with maternal age | | |
| Clarifies the vast majority are not inherited, therefore no increased risk in future pregnancy | | |
| Discusses physical features of Down's Syndrome | | |
| Discusses effect on developmental delay | | |
| Discusses congenital abnormalities associated with Down's Syndrome | | |
| Discusses prognosis and life expectancy | | |
| Discusses options to continue or terminate pregnancy | | |
| Explains procedure for TOP at 17 weeks | | |
| | | |
| Identifies patient's ideas, concerns and expectations in an empathetic manner | | |
| Summarises key points, checks understanding & avoids jargon | | |
| Suggests follow up or take home information | | |
| Completes station in a confident and professional manner | | |
| | | |
| Examiners Global Mark | /5 | |
| Actors Global Mark | /5 | |
| Total Station Mark | /30 | |

# Learning points

- There are two methods of screening for Down's syndrome: serum screening and ultrasound screening (nuchal translucency). These can be used in combination (the combined test) up to 14 weeks gestation.

- Common physical features of Down's syndrome include facial characteristics (e.g. large protruding tongue, slanted eyes, narrow roof of mouth, flattened head and nose, low set ears), single palmar crease and 'sandal gap' separation of $1^{st}$ and $2^{nd}$ toes.

- Congenital heart defects are found in almost 1 in 2 children with Down's syndrome. The most common defects include a atrioventricular or ventricular septal defect (80%), Tetralogy of Fallot or patent ductus arteriosus.

# Station 43: Intrauterine Growth Restriction

## Candidate Instructions

You are the Foundation Year Doctor in the Antenatal Clinic. You have been asked to speak to Anisha, a 29-year-old pregnant woman who has come in following her 20 week scan. She has been told that her baby is small for gestational age and this is under investigation. She wants to find out more information about what this means for her baby and how this will be investigated or monitored.

Please answer any questions or concerns she may have.

You do not need to examine the patient.

You have eight minutes

## Actor Instructions

You are Anisha, a 29-year-old Pharmacist and you are 20 weeks pregnant with your first child. You have come to the Antenatal Clinic following your 20-week scan after you were told your baby is small for their dates. You wanted to ask some questions about what this means and how it will affect you and your baby.

This is your first pregnancy and has otherwise been unremarkable. You noticed you have not got a very big bump but just put this down to the fact that you and your partner are both quite 'small-made'.

Apart from anaemia for which you take iron tablets, you feel well and have had no recent fevers or infections. Before pregnancy, you were underweight and scarcely had periods, which is why you were surprised when you finally did get pregnant after 2 years.

You reluctantly admit to the doctor that you currently smoke 5 cigarettes/day, which is much lower than what you were smoking before pregnancy (20/day) but feel you need this has you have smoked for such a long time.

Questions you would like to ask if the doctor:

- What can cause the baby to be small?
- Could this all just be because my husband and I are both 'small-made'?
- Do you think this is because I have been smoking while pregnant?
- What will happen now – will there be more investigations/scans?
- Will I still be able to have a normal delivery?
- What are the risks of having a small baby?
- Could my baby die

## Examiner Instructions

The candidate is a Foundation Year Doctor in the Antenatal Clinic. They have been asked to speak to Anisha, a 29-year-old pregnant woman, who has come in following her 20 week scan. She has been told that her baby is small for gestational age and this is under investigation. She wants to find out more information about what this means for her baby and how this will be investigated or monitored.

They have been asked to discuss any concerns she may have.

They do not need to examine the patient.

## Mark Scheme

| Task | Achieved | Not Achieved |
|---|---|---|
| Introduces self, washes hands | | |
| Confirms name, age & occupation of patient | | |
| Establishes reason for consultation | | |
| | | |
| Clarifies patient's current knowledge base | | |
| Discusses physiological causes for a baby to be small for dates (steady growth but small) | | |
| Discuss pathological causes of small-for-dates foetus (i.e. IUGR) | | |
| Takes brief history to elicit possible risk factors (e.g. smoking, low maternal weight) | | |
| Discusses further maternal investigations to check for medical conditions or infections | | |
| Discusses investigating blood flow (Doppler USS) | | |
| Discusses possible invasive testing for karyotyping or infection screen | | |
| Discusses investigations to check health of baby - CTG | | |
| Explains that she will continue to be monitored in secondary care | | |
| Explains that IUGR may lead to premature delivery if compromised fetus | | |
| Sensitively explains that there may be an increased risk of stillbirth or neonatal death | | |
| Advice given re: smoking cessation | | |
| Safety netting – to return if any concerns including pain, bleeding or feeling unwell | | |
| | | |
| Identifies patient's ideas, concerns and expectations in an empathetic manner | | |
| Summarises key points, checks understanding & avoids jargon | | |
| Suggests follow up or take home information | | |
| Completes station in a confident and professional manner | | |
| | | |
| Examiners Global Mark | /5 | |
| Actors Global Mark | /5 | |
| Total Station Mark | /30 | |

## Learning points

- A small for gestational age fetus can either be physiological or pathological. Keep in mind the centiles used span across the whole population and are not altered for patients with different ethnicities or medical backgrounds. Inevitably, some will just be small but growing steadily.

- Maternal disease, smoking, drugs, diet and infection, as well as congenital abnormalities can all cause IUGR.

- It is important to document serial measurements of fundal height to differentiate between growth restriction and a small fetus.

# Station 44: Pain Relief in Pregnancy

## Candidate Instructions

You are the Foundation Year Doctor in the Antenatal clinic. You have been asked to see Amy, a 32-year-old woman who is 28 weeks pregnant. She wishes to ask you about pain relief options in labour. Please discuss the options available to her and answer any questions she may have.

You do not need to examine the patient.

You have eight minutes.

## Actor Instructions

You are Amy, a 32-year-old phlebotomist. You have presented to the Antenatal clinic today to ask questions about pain relief options in labour. You are currently 28 weeks pregnant with your first baby.

Ultimately, you would like to have as little intervention as possible, but you are scared that you will change your mind at the last minute and would like to know your options.

You have heard about conservative methods including the exercise ball, baths, aromatherapy and massage, which you are willing to try. You have been attending NCT classes with your husband to practice breathing exercises, and he will be with you in the delivery room.

You are keen to know how effective the TENs machine is as you are considering investing in one. You have also heard about gas and air, but heard from someone in your NCT class this can make you feel sick.

You have been considering an epidural but you are fearful of the idea of a needle in your spine, and are scared you will not be able to move your legs or feel anything, thereby affecting the progression of your labour. You are also scared about whether it would affect the baby. You are also interested in the complications of the procedure and if there can be any long term effects.

You are otherwise fit and well. You have had no other pregnancies. The current pregnancy has been uncomplicated and you are planning to give birth in the midwife-led centre, but are prepared to move to the labour ward if the need arises.

## Examiner Instructions

The candidate is a Foundation Year Doctor in the Antenatal clinic. They have been asked to see Amy, a 32-year-old woman who is 28 weeks pregnant. She wishes to ask about pain relief options in labour. The candidate has been asked to discuss the options available and answer any questions she may have.

They do not need to examine the patient.

**Mark Scheme**

| Task | Achieved | Not Achieved |
|---|---|---|
| Introduces self, washes hands | | |
| Confirms name, age & occupation of patient | | |
| Establishes reason for consultation | | |
| Identifies current knowledge of available options and preferences expressed | | |
| Asks if mother is attending antenatal classes providing support and information | | |
| Asks if she has support or birthing partner | | |
| Discusses non-medical options, breathing exercises | | |
| Remains non-judgemental and unbiased when alternative therapies are discussed | | |
| Discusses TENS machine (transcutaneous electrical nerve stimulation) | | |
| Discusses gas & air/Entonox – mild analgesia | | |
| Discusses Pethidine IM injection – moderate analgesia, discusses side effects & cautions | | |
| Side effects: sedation, nausea, respiratory depression if given too late in labour | | |
| Discusses how epidural analgesia is administered and its effect | | |
| Discusses advantages of epidural | | |
| Discusses disadvantages and increased risks associated with epidural | | |
| Discusses option of spinal anaesthetic (strong analgesia with loss of function, also used for caesarean section)) | | |
| | | |
| Identifies patient's ideas, concerns and expectations in an empathetic manner | | |
| Summarises key points, checks understanding & avoids jargon | | |
| Suggests follow up or take home information | | |
| Completes station in a confident and professional manner | | |
| | | |
| Examiners Global Mark | /5 | |
| Actors Global Mark | /5 | |
| Total Station Mark | /30 | |

## Learning points

- There are many alternative therapies available for women in labour, including hypnotherapy, aromatherapy, TENS machines and acupuncture. As a doctor it is important to clarify what is researched based and what is anecdotal. Equally, some mothers may find these methods very effective, so it is important not to dismiss this or be judgemental about their preferences.

- It is important to reassure the patient, emphasise patient choice and invite the patient to talk about any specific worries or concerns she may have. Birth plans can be created with not only one option but escalating options depending upon how circumstances evolve.

- Some basic knowledge around epidurals is important to give a solid overview of this option. Epidural analgesia is a central nerve block technique providing complete relief in 95% of cases and reducing need for further analgesia if forceps, vacuum or caesarean section are required. Disadvantages include transient hypotension and increasing the duration of the second stage of labour.

# Station 45: Counselling following Intrauterine death

## Candidate Instructions

You are the Foundation Year Doctor on the delivery unit. You have been asked to see Perrie, a 28-year-old woman who has been admitted to the delivery suite 'Butterfly Room' after discovering yesterday that she has lost her baby at 30 weeks. The consultant has explained this to her and she is due to be induced today as requested.

You were asked to cannulate the patient, but before you begin, she asks to speak to you. Please answer any questions she may have.

You do not need to examine the patient.

You have eight minutes.

## Actor Instructions

You are Perrie, a 28-year-old call handler. You have presented to the delivery suite today for induction of labour after discovering that your unborn baby had died yesterday. The junior doctor on the ward has been asked to take bloods from you but you asked to speak to them to ask a few questions about what to expect today.

You noted reduced movements over the past few days and yesterday could not feel any movements and so presented to the maternity unit, where you were informed by the consultant that the baby had died. You and your partner are still in shock and trying to process what has happened. You had a long discussion with the consultant yesterday, but did not feel ready to ask questions. More importantly, you are keen to get this over with because it is very upsetting to still have the baby in your tummy, and so requested to be induced today.

Your partner and family have been very supportive but everyone is understandably very upset by the news.

This is your second pregnancy. Your first child – a boy – is now 3 years old. He has no idea what is going on and has been excited to have a little brother or sister.

Questions you would like to ask the doctor:

- What will happen now? I remember the consultant said they would place a tablet inside my vagina, but how long will the process take?
- What will happen to the baby? Will I get to see them?
- Will we be able to find out what caused this after the baby is born?
- Why did this happen? Could I have prevented this?
- Will this stop me having any other children?

# Examiner Instructions

The candidate is a Foundation Year Doctor on the delivery unit. They have been asked to see Perrie, a 28-year-old woman who has been admitted to the delivery suite 'Butterfly Room' after discovering yesterday that she has lost her baby at 30 weeks. The consultant has explained this to her and she is due to be induced today as requested.

The candidate was asked to cannulate the patient, but before they begin, Perrie has asked to speak to them. The candidate has been asked to answer any questions she may have.

They do not need to examine the patient.

**Mark Scheme**

| Task | Achieved | Not Achieved |
|---|---|---|
| Introduces self, washes hands | | |
| Confirms name, age & occupation of patient | | |
| Establishes reason for discussion | | |
| | | |
| Expresses sympathy for loss of baby | | |
| Takes brief history of events leading up to death | | |
| Asks about how patient feels about the news | | |
| Establishes support network and if coping | | |
| Allows periods of silence and active listening | | |
| Clarifies what patient understands or remembers from consultant discussion | | |
| Explains the process of induction to mother | | |
| Explains that they can be given time after to spend with baby and hold baby if they wish | | |
| Explains that tests/post mortem can be done to try to find the cause of the intrauterine death if they wish | | |
| Details common causes of intrauterine death | | |
| Stresses that intrauterine deaths are most commonly not preventable | | |
| Explains further pregnancies are unlikely to be affected by intrauterine death | | |
| Checks if happy to go ahead with induction today | | |
| | | |
| Identifies patient's ideas, concerns and expectations in an empathetic manner | | |
| Summarises key points, checks understanding & avoids jargon | | |
| Suggests follow up or take home information about support groups or counselling | | |
| Completes station in a confident and professional manner | | |
| | | |
| Examiners Global Mark | /5 | |
| Actors Global Mark | /5 | |
| Total Station Mark | /30 | |

## Learning points

- Where the death of the baby is diagnosed antenatally, labour is induced using prostaglandins administered vaginally. This does not need to be immediate, but should happen within 2-3 days.

- In many cases, the cause of intrauterine death is unknown, which can be very distressing for the patient. IUGR, congenital abnormalities or placental complications can otherwise cause intrauterine death.

- This is a difficult and emotive scenario to handle, and you would not be expected to break this news at medical student level, but may unexpectedly be asked questions as you are present on the ward. Compassion and communication skills are needed as much as, if not more than, knowledge base when faced with this scenario in real life or the OSCE. "The quality of care that bereaved families receive when their baby dies has long-lasting effects. Good care cannot remove parents' pain and grief, but poor care can and does make things much worse - 'Stillbirth And Neonatal Death Society' (SANDS)

# Ethics & Law

## Station 46: Fraser Guidelines – Contraceptive Advice in Underage Teens

### Candidate Instructions

You are the Foundation Year Doctor in a GP surgery. Lucille is a 15-year-old girl who has come in to discuss contraception. Please counsel the patient in view of her age and determine her suitability for receiving contraceptive advice. You do not need to counsel her about a specific type of contraception – this is not tested as part of the scenario.

You do not need to examine the patient.

You have eight minutes.

## Actor Instructions

You are Lucille, a 15-year-old schoolgirl. You have come to see the GP today as you would like to discuss contraception.

You have been with your current boyfriend for the past 2 years, and you recently started to have intercourse. Given that you are terrified of getting pregnant, you researched alternative contraceptive methods to using condoms.

The candidate will need to ask you questions about your relationship in order to ensure that you are safe in the relationship. Your partner is also 15 years old, and he is in your class at school. The decision to start having sex was mutual, and you do not feel pressured at all.

You absolutely do not want to discuss this with your parents as they will freak out as they are very religious and only believe in sex after marriage. You are scared they may tell his parents to stop you seeing him or tell the school and everyone will find out. You are worried about it getting around school because you do not want to be labelled as a 'slag'. You want the doctor to promise you that they will not tell your parents.

Even if you do not get contraception from the doctor, you will still continue having sex with your boyfriend, but you are always anxious about the risk of getting pregnant.

You have been thinking about starting the pill but want to know more about your options, and you would like some information that you can go away and think about.

## Examiner Instructions

The candidate is a Foundation Year Doctor in a GP surgery. Lucille is a 15-year-old girl who has come in to discuss contraception. They have been asked to counsel the patient in view of her age and determine her suitability for receiving contraceptive advice. They do not need to counsel the patient about a specific type of contraception – this is not tested as part of the scenario.

They do not need to examine the patient.

**Mark Scheme**

| Task | Achieved | Not Achieved |
|---|---|---|
| Introduces self, washes hands | | |
| Confirms name & age of patient | | |
| Establishes reason for consultation | | |
| | | |
| Gives warning shot re: sensitive questions and reiterates confidentiality | | |
| Establishes if patient is currently sexually active | | |
| Establishes age of current sexual partner | | |
| Establishes whether concerns over child safety or coercion at present | | |
| Enquires about current contraceptive use | | |
| Establishes that patient will continue to be sexually active without contraceptive advice | | |
| Asks if she has discussed this with her parents | | |
| Discusses concerns surrounding telling her parents | | |
| Encourages patient to discuss with parents (as per Fraser guidelines) | | |
| Reassures patient that they have a right to confidentiality | | |
| Sensitively advises confidentially only broken in times of concern for safety | | |
| Determines whether they should give patient contraceptive advice | | |
| Discusses patient's current knowledge of contraceptive options | | |
| | | |
| Identifies patient's ideas, concerns and expectations in an empathetic manner | | |
| Summarises key points, checks understanding & avoids jargon | | |
| Suggests follow up or take home information | | |
| Completes station in a confident and professional manner | | |
| | | |
| Examiners Global Mark | /5 | |
| Actors Global Mark | /5 | |
| Total Station Mark | /30 | |

## Learning points

- Contraceptive advice to underage teens (under 16) can present an array of ethical dilemmas. Remember to address each issue; is the patient Gillick competent? Do they fulfill Fraser guidelines? Is there a child safety concern? Does confidentiality need to be breached?

- Remember not to confuse Gillick competence with Fraser guidelines! Gillick competence relates to **any** decision that a young person is asked to make, and only relates to their ability to consent to (and not refuse) treatment. Fraser guidelines relate to contraception/abortion advice **only**.

- Issues with confidentiality are extremely important to young people, and the GMC state that we should maintain confidentiality whenever possible, without allowing harm to come to a child/young person. This is essential in ensuring young people engage with services. Be sure to stress this to your patients, but also make them aware when you are concerned.

## Station 47: Conscientious Objection

## Candidate Instructions

You are the Foundation Year Doctor at a GP surgery. Terry is a medical student based at your surgery. At the end of your clinic, he asks to discuss the issue of conscientious objection, having observed a consultation between one of the other GPs and a young woman requesting a termination.

Please answer any questions they may have.

You have eight minutes.

## Actor Instructions

You are Terry, a fifth year medical student on placement in a GP surgery. You have been shadowing one of the other GPs today, and observed them discussing termination of pregnancy with a young woman. You would like to discuss how conscientious objection works in practise. You have approached the candidate, a Foundation Year Doctor at the surgery, to discuss this as you feel more comfortable talking to a near-peer.

Due to your religious beliefs, you do not feel termination of pregnancy is morally correct, and therefore feel uncomfortable with the idea of participating in providing this service to women. You also believe that extra-marital sex is wrong.

You would like to ask the following questions:

- In the UK, is a doctor legally allowed to refuse to offer a service such as termination on the basis of conscientious objection?
- When conscientiously objecting to termination, would a doctor have to explain anything to the patient?
- What happens if the employer makes termination of pregnancy a service that all doctors are contractually obliged to offer?
- Is it possible to offer termination services to only certain patients? For example, if the pregnancy was due to sexual assault, or only participating in termination involving married couples?
- What is the policy if I am permitted to conscientiously object in my workplace, but a patient comes in to A&E with a complication to termination? Would I have to be involved?

## Examiner Instructions

The candidate is a Foundation Year Doctor in a GP surgery. Terry is a medical student based at their surgery. At the end of their clinic, Terry asks to discuss the issue of conscientious objection, having observed a consultation between one of the other GPs and a young woman requesting a termination. The candidate has been asked to answer any questions they may have.

## Mark Scheme

| Task | Achieved | Not Achieved |
|---|---|---|
| Introduces self, washes hands | | |
| Confirms name and year of clinical study | | |
| Establishes reason for discussion | | |
| | | |
| Sensitively asks student what their conscientious objection relates to and their beliefs | | |
| Explains doctors can object to participate in certain treatments in UK based on their beliefs | | |
| Explains that GMC states that the care of the patient must always remain the priority | | |
| Emphasises that a patient must not come to harm due to the doctor's beliefs | | |
| Explains that the reason for conscientious objection does not need to be fully disclosed | | |
| Explains that the doctor should behave in a non-judgemental manner | | |
| Explains contractual obligations must be fulfilled | | |
| Explains that any contractual dispute with the hospital/employer needs to be resolved locally | | |
| Advises that situations should be highlighted early and discussed with a consultant | | |
| Explains GMC states colleagues should not be over-burdened due to a colleague's objection | | |
| Explains that it is discriminatory to only offer certain treatments to select patients based on their lifestyle choices | | |
| Explains that all doctors have a duty of care to manage acutely unwell patients | | |
| Identifies student's ideas, concerns and expectations in an empathetic manner | | |
| Summarises key points, checks understanding & avoids jargon | | |
| Offers take home information | | |
| Completes station in a confident and professional manner | | |
| | | |
| Examiners Global Mark | /5 | |
| Actors Global Mark | /5 | |
| Total Station Mark | /30 | |

## Learning points

- It is important for all specialities to be aware of the GMC Duties of a Doctor guidance, as this scenario touches on some key issues surrounding conscientious objection.

- Doctors may practise medicine in accordance with their beliefs, provided that they act in accordance with relevant legislation and do not treat patients unfairly, do not deny patients access to appropriate medical treatment or services and do not cause patients distress.

- The GMC states that if a clinician has personal views that will preclude them from seeing or treating particular patients they must make this clear to their employers as early as possible to mitigate delays or risk to patients. The doctor's wishes should also be respected but the wider impact on patients and services also needs to be considered and allowed for.

## Station 48: Female Genital Mutilation

## Candidate Instructions

You are the Foundation Year Doctor on the Obstetrics team. One of the women in labour is known to have had FGM performed on her as a child. Diana, the medical student attached to the team, would like to speak with you to understand more about the legal responsibilities of healthcare professionals in dealing with cases of FGM.

Please answer any questions they may have.

You have eight minutes.

## Actor Instructions

You are Diana, a fourth year medical student currently on your attachment with the Obstetric team on Labour Ward. During the morning ward round, you joined the team in reviewing a mother in labour who is known to have had FGM performed on her as a child. This is the first case of FGM that you have ever seen, and you have some questions about the legal responsibilities of healthcare professionals when dealing with such cases. You are aware that all forms of FGM are illegal in the UK.

You have some questions to ask the Foundation Year doctor on Labour Ward today. These questions will help to direct the conversation:

- I have heard that there is mandatory reporting in certain cases of FGM. What are the situations where a healthcare professional would have a legal responsibility to report this?
- What happens if the patient refuses to give consent to report her case?
- What information needs to be recorded when seeing a woman with a confirmed history of FGM?
- What if the patient or her partner asks you to repair the scar?
- I have seen some women having an episiotomy during their deliveries. Does this count as FGM?

## Examiner Instructions

The candidate is a Foundation Year Doctor on the Obstetrics team. One of the women in labour is known to have had FGM performed on her as a child. Diana, the medical student attached to the team, would like to speak with the candidate to understand more about the legal responsibilities of healthcare professionals in dealing with cases of FGM. The candidate has been asked to answer any questions they may have.

**Mark Scheme**

| Task | Achieved | Not Achieved |
|---|---|---|
| Introduces self, washes hands | | |
| Confirms name and year of clinical study | | |
| Establishes reason for discussion | | |
| Identifies student's current knowledge base regarding FGM reporting | | |
| Defines FGM | | |
| Explains mandatory reporting for anyone <18 years of age with confirmed/suspected FGM | | |
| Explains that any child/young person suspected of being at risk of having FGM must be reported | | |
| Explains that it is not a mandatory requirement to report all pregnant women with FGM | | |
| Explains pregnant mother whose unborn child is deemed to be at risk of FGM must be reported | | |
| Explains there is no legal requirement to report woman aged ≥ 18 if not deemed to be at risk | | |
| Explains reporting FGM in a child/child at risk must be done even without parental consent | | |
| Explains if a competent adult at risk refuses consent to reporting, we must respect this | | |
| Explains that the type of FGM should be clearly documented using the WHO classification | | |
| Explains FGM must be documented in the notes in all cases, even if it is not the reason for review | | |
| Explains that re-suturing FGM scar tissue is illegal under UK law (re-infibulation) | | |
| Explains that re-infibulation will not be undertaken under any circumstance | | |
| Explains that an episiotomy is not classified as FGM as it is a required surgical procedure | | |
| | | |
| Summarises key points, checks understanding | | |
| Offers take home information | | |
| Completes station in a confident and professional manner | | |
| | | |
| Examiners Global Mark | /5 | |
| Actors Global Mark | /5 | |
| Total Station Mark | /30 | |

## Learning points

- Doctors and healthcare professionals have a **legal** duty to report cases of FGM in young females under the age of 18 in all circumstances, whether consent has been obtained or not

- FGM refers to the total or partial removal of female genitalia for **non-medical** reasons. The WHO classification allows doctors to stratify the level of injury:

Type 1: Often referred to as clitoridectomy, this is the partial or total removal of the clitoris
Type 2: Often referred to as excision, this is the partial or total removal of the clitoris and the labia minora
Type 3: Often referred to as infibulation, this is the narrowing of the vaginal opening through the creation of a covering seal. The seal is formed by cutting and repositioning the labia minora
Type 4: This includes all other harmful procedures to the female genitalia for non-medical purposes, e.g. pricking, piercing, incising, scraping and cauterizing the genital area

- This is a very difficult station and is an evolving topic. Make sure you know the difference between the national guidance (which is currently the Royal College of Obstetrics and Gynaecology (RCOG) "green top" guideline), which may differ from locally made policies

# Station 49: Paternal Rights

## Candidate Instructions

You are the Foundation Year Doctor on the Obstetrics team. One of your patients is in active labour but is not progressing well. Your registrar has suggested that an emergency caesarean section may be required to deliver the baby safely if things do not progress quickly in the next 30 minutes. However, the patient has firmly stated that she does not wish to have a caesarean under any circumstances. Her husband has asked to speak to a member of the team. Your registrar has asked you to speak with her husband, Colin, and answer any questions that he may have.

Please answer any questions they may have.

You have eight minutes.

## Actor Instructions

You are Colin, the husband of one of the patients on the Obstetric Ward. Your wife is currently in active labour. She started having contractions a long time ago and you thought that the baby would have been delivered by now. The Obstetric team have been observing her closely, and have stated that they feel the labour is not progressing as well as they would like. As a result, the registrar suggested that an emergency caesarean section may be required in order to deliver the baby if the situation does not improve within 30 minutes.

Your wife was very upset at the mention of a caesarean section, as she desperately wants to have a normal delivery. This is your first child and you both have heard stories of the complications of women who underwent caesarean section. However, whilst you feel the team should do whatever is safest for the baby, your wife stated that she would not consent to a caesarean section.

You have asked to speak a member of the obstetric team to ask some questions as to your rights in this situation. You understand the medical reasons why the doctors have raised the possibility of requiring an emergency caesarean section, and you are worried that your wife will regret her decision should anything happen to the baby.

How do the team decide if my wife is in a suitable state to give consent to a procedure?

She has already said that she does not want to have an emergency caesarean section. Does this mean that this is no longer an option as she has stated that she would not consent?

What happens if, after reassessing my wife, she still refuses to have a caesarean section? What will the team do then?

What would happen in the scenario that my wife refuses to consent for a caesarean section, but the life of our baby is at risk?

Would it be possible for me to consent on my wife's behalf if she refuses? What rights do I have at this stage as the father?

# Examiner Instructions

The candidate is a Foundation Year Doctor on the Obstetrics team. One of the ward patients is in active labour but is not progressing well. The registrar has suggested that an emergency caesarean section may be required to deliver the baby safely if things do not progress quickly in the next 30 minutes. However, the patient has firmly stated that she does not wish to have a caesarean under any circumstances. Her husband has asked to speak to a member of the team.

The registrar has asked the candidate to speak with her husband, Colin, and answer any questions that he may have.

**Mark Scheme**

| Task | Achieved | Not Achieved |
|---|---|---|
| Introduces self, washes hands | | |
| Confirms name and relation to patient | | |
| Establishes reason for discussion | | |
| | | |
| Identifies husband's current understanding of the situation | | |
| Elicits husband's concerns for mother and baby | | |
| Explains that several factors are considered in determining one's ability to make a decision | | |
| Explains that capacity to make a decision is based on an individual being able to understand and retain information provided | | |
| Explains that an individual must be able to weigh up the pros and cons of treatment | | |
| Explains that an individual must be able to communicate their decision | | |
| Explains that adults are assumed to be able to make these decisions unless there is reason to suspect that this ability may be impaired | | |
| Explains that the decision must be informed and non-coerced in order to be valid | | |
| Explains that the child has no rights until birth | | |
| Explains that if the baby was at risk, doctors cannot intervene without maternal consent | | |
| Explains that a relative cannot make a decision on behalf of an adult if they have capacity | | |
| Explains under UK law, there are no paternal rights in this case | | |
| Suggests husband raises concerns with his wife | | |
| Offers to have discussion with couple with senior during next review | | |
| Summarises key points, checks understanding | | |
| Offers take home information | | |
| Completes station in a confident and professional manner | | |
| | | |
| Examiners Global Mark | /5 | |
| Actors Global Mark | /5 | |
| Total Station Mark | /30 | |

## Learning points

- Autonomy is one of the fundamental principles in medical ethics. All healthcare professionals must work to uphold the autonomy of their patients wherever possible.

- Relatives cannot consent for patients, whether or not they currently have capacity. It is important to make it clear that if they do not have capacity, the decision is made by the team, often taking into consideration the viewpoint of their relatives.

- The foetus/baby does not have any legal rights until after birth. Legally, the unborn baby is seen as being a part of the mother, and therefore she has complete autonomy over the child.

# Station 50: Domestic Violence in Pregnancy

## Candidate Instructions

You are the Foundation Year Doctor in a GP practice. You have been asked to speak to 19-year-old Jeannie, who is 12 weeks pregnant with her first baby. She has booked into to see you today following her booking visit with the midwife. The midwife has asked you to see her because she is concerned about her mood. Please discuss her concerns.

You do not need to examine the patient

You have eight minutes

## Actor Instructions

You are Jeannie, a 19-year-old hairdresser. You have just been to see the midwife for your booking visit and she asked you to wait to see the doctor. You became quite tearful when she started discussing your support network. You are feeling low, but state it is because of stress at home. You do not want to cause any trouble and make a 'big deal' out of nothing.

You are currently 12 weeks pregnant with your first baby with your boyfriend of 2 years, Marcus, a mechanic. It was not planned, although you have decided to keep it after discussion with your boyfriend.

Currently, you are living with your mum and your boyfriend lives nearby. He is keen for you to move in with him and his mum but you are reluctant because of relationship issues.

In the past few weeks since finding out you were pregnant, you have been having more heated arguments with Marcus, mainly about the living situation and money issues. Last week, you brought up the issue of how you were going to split the costs when buying stuff for the baby, and he snapped and called you a 'gold-digger'. You were very hurt, but you know he's stressed about how you are going to afford everything and he is trying to make ends meet.

Two days ago, you found another girl's number in his recent text messages and you started screaming at him, even though he was drunk. He tends to binge drink at weekends with his friends, which coincides with when you have your biggest fights. You know you were in the wrong for doing so and the argument escalated and Marcus shoved you to get out of the way as he walked out. You fell, and he apologised profusely and you forgave him, but you were in shock because it was the first time it has ever got physical.

You do not want to get him in trouble because you love him and you are sure he is going to be an amazing father but the pregnancy has put a lot of stress on the relationship. You have not told anyone what happened because you were not harmed and you do not want people to think badly of him. You do not want to report him to the police as you do not see this as 'abuse', and you do not want him to find out you have discussed this.

## Examiner Instructions

The candidate is a Foundation Year Doctor in a GP practice. They have been asked to speak to 19-year-old Jeannie, who is 12 weeks pregnant with her first baby. She has booked into today following her booking visit with the midwife. The midwife has asked the candidate to see Jeannie because she is concerned about her mood. They have been asked to discuss her concerns.

They do not need to examine the patient.

## Mark Scheme

| Task | Achieved | Not Achieved |
|---|---|---|
| Introduces self, washes hands | | |
| Confirms name, age & occupation | | |
| Establishes reason for consultation | | |
| Allows patient to discuss mood and concerns with relationship | | |
| Directly asks about physical or verbal abuse or acts causing harm | | |
| Checks if patient sustained any injuries during physical encounter | | |
| Asks patient if she wishes to remain with partner – maintains non-judgemental approach | | |
| Highlights that 30% abuse starts in pregnancy | | |
| Discuss different types of abuse and examples of what this includes | | |
| Discuss risks to unborn baby – miscarriage, prematurity, death or injury | | |
| Discuss if ongoing risk to unborn child would need to inform social services, ideally with patient's consent | | |
| Discuss living situation – highlight concerns about moving in with partner | | |
| Encourage patient to tell family member/friend to discuss and for support | | |
| Discuss safety plan if feels unsafe or if situation escalates | | |
| Encourage to visit if any physical injuries and importance of photographing these | | |
| Advise patient to call 999 if in imminent danger | | |
| Remains non-judgemental of patient's choice | | |
| | | |
| Summarises key points, checks understanding | | |
| Suggests follow up or take home information (e.g. helpline, contact for support groups) | | |
| Completes station in a confident and professional manner | | |
| | | |
| Examiners Global Mark | /5 | |
| Actors Global Mark | /5 | |
| Total Station Mark | /30 | |

## Learning points

- Domestic abuse in pregnancy is more common than you think – always remember to ask a detailed social history and to ask about relationships and support in pregnancy.

- Remember – you cannot force someone to tell the police. You can only break confidentiality if there is imminent danger to the patient or the public.

- However, if there are children involved in the same household as the domestic abuse, you have an absolute duty of care to inform social services even without the parent's consent.

# References

BNF. (Oct 2016). *Hormone replacement therapy.* Available:
https://www.evidence.nhs.uk/formulary/bnf/current/6-endocrine-system/64-sex-hormones/641-female-sex-hormones-and-their-modulators/6411-oestrogens-and-hrt/hormone-replacement-therapy. Last accessed 4th Nov 2016.

Burgio KL, Borello-France D, Richter HE, et al; Risk factors for fecal and urinary incontinence after childbirth: the childbirth and pelvic symptoms study. Am J Gastroenterol. 2007 Sep;102(9):1998-2004. Epub 2007 Jun 15

CDC. (2003). *Exposure to Blood: What Healthcare Personnel Need to Know.* Available:
http://www.cdc.gov/hai/pdfs/bbp/exp_to_blood.pdf. Last accessed 4th Nov 2016.

Donegan, K., King, B., Bryan, P. Safety of pertussis vaccination in pregnant women in UK: observational study. *BMJ* 2014:349:g4219

Faculty of Sexual & Reproductive Healthcare (FSRH) (2014). *Venous Thromboembolism (VTE) and Hormonal Contraception.* Available:
www.fsrh.org/documents/fsrhstatementvteandhormonalcontraception-november/fsrhstatementvteandhormonalcontraception-november.pdf+&cd=3&hl=en&ct=clnk&gl=uk. Last accessed 4th Nov 2016.

HFEA. (1990). *Human Fertilisation and Embryology Act 1990.*Available:
http://www.legislation.gov.uk/ukpga/1990/37/crossheading/abortion. Last accessed 4th Nov 2016.

Impey, L. Child, T. (2012). Disorders of Early Pregnancy. In: Impey, L. Child, T. *Obstetrics & Gynaecology.* 4th ed. London: Wiley-Blackwell. p118-128.

Kirk E, Bottomley C, Bourne T. (2013). Diagnosing ectopic pregnancy and current concepts in the management of pregnancy of unknown location.. *Human Reproduction Update.* 20 (2), p250-261.

Nair M & Knight M., Maternal Mortality in the UK 2011-13: Surveillance and Epidemiology Manisha Nair and Marian Knight. In Knight M, Tuffnell D, Kenyon S, Shakespeare J, Gray R, Kurinczuk JJ (Eds.) on behalf of MBRRACE-UK. Saving Lives, Improving Mothers' Care - Surveillance of maternal deaths in the UK 2011-13 and lessons learned to inform maternity care from the UK and Ireland Confidential Enquiries into Maternal Deaths and Morbidity 2009-13. Oxford: National Perinatal Epidemiology Unit, University of Oxford 2015: p7-21.

NICE (Aug 2016). *Fertility problems: assessment and treatment [CG156].*Available:
https://www.nice.org.uk/guidance/cg156/uptake. Last accessed 4th Nov 2016.

NICE (Sept 2016). *Care in third stage of labour.* Available:
http://pathways.nice.org.uk/pathways/intrapartum-care#path=view%3A/pathways/intrapartum-care/care-in-third-stage-of-labour.xml&content=view-quality-statement%3Aquality-statements-delayed-cord-clamping. Last accessed 4th Nov 2016.

Nwokolo, N., Dragovic, B., Patel, S., Tong, C., Barker, G., Radcliffe, K.. (2016). 2015 UK national guideline for the management of infection with Chlamydia trachomatis. *International Journal of STD & AIDS.* 27 (4), p251–267.

Public Health England. (2015). *Cervical screening: programme overview.* Available:
https://www.gov.uk/guidance/cervical-screening-programme-overview. Last accessed 4th Nov 2016.

Qureshi, H., Massey, E., Kirwan, D., Davies, T., Robson, S., White, J., Jones, J. and Allard, S. (2014), BCSH guideline for the use of anti-D immunoglobulin for the prevention of haemolytic disease of the fetus and newborn. Transfusion Med, 24: 8–20. doi:10.1111/tme.12091

Rotterdam ESHRE/ASRM-Sponsored PCOS Consensus Workshop Group. (2003). Revised 2003 consensus on diagnostic criteria and long-term health risks related to polycystic ovary syndrome. *Fertility & Sterility. American Society for Reproductive Medicine.* 81 (1), 0015-0282.

Royal College of Obstetricians and Gynaecologists (RCOG). (2008). *Chickenpox in pregnancy: what you need to know.*Available: https://www.rcog.org.uk/globalassets/documents/patients/patient-information-leaflets/pregnancy/chickenpox-in-pregnancy.pdf. Last accessed 4th Nov 2016.

Royal College of Obstetricians and Gynaecologists (RCOG). (2013).*Heavy bleeding after birth (postpartum haemorrhage).* Available: https://www.rcog.org.uk/globalassets/documents/patients/patient-information-leaflets/pregnancy/heavy-bleeding-after-birth.pdf. Last accessed 4th Nov 2016.

Printed in Great Britain
by Amazon

62449061R00159